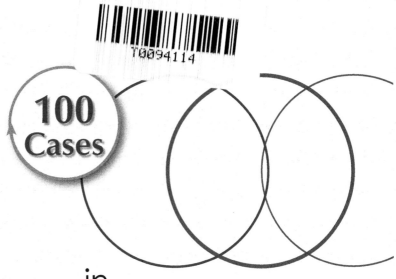

100 Cases

in
Clinical
Pharmacology,
Therapeutics
and Prescribing

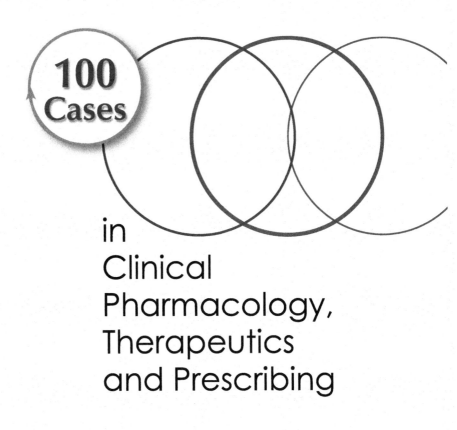

100 Cases

in Clinical Pharmacology, Therapeutics and Prescribing

Kerry Layne MBBS, BSc (Hons), PhD, MRCP
Specialist Registrar in Clinical Pharmacology
and Therapeutics/General Medicine, Guy's and St Thomas' NHS
Foundation Trust, London, UK

Albert Ferro PhD, FRCP, FBPhS, FBIHS, FESC
Professor of Cardiovascular Clinical Pharmacology, King's College
London, and Honorary Consultant Physician, Guy's
and St Thomas' NHS Foundation Trust, London, UK

100 Cases Series Editor:
Janice Rymer MBBS, FRACP
Professor of Obstetrics & Gynaecology and Dean of Student Affairs,
King's College London School of Medicine, London, UK

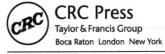
CRC Press
Taylor & Francis Group
Boca Raton London New York

CRC Press is an imprint of the
Taylor & Francis Group, an **Informa** business

CRC Press
Taylor & Francis Group
6000 Broken Sound Parkway NW, Suite 300
Boca Raton, FL 33487-2742

© 2020 by Taylor & Francis Group, LLC
CRC Press is an imprint of Taylor & Francis Group, an Informa business

No claim to original U.S. Government works

International Standard Book Number-13: 978-1-138-48967-7 (Hardback)
978-1-138-48959-2 (Paperback)

CONTENTS

PREFACE

Clinical pharmacology is the study of drug use in humans. It is closely linked to therapeutics, which is the study of how diseases are treated. A good understanding of both subjects is essential for safe and effective prescribing, either by doctors or by the more recent (and rapidly increasing) generation of non-medical prescribers.

Drugs of one sort or another have been used by physicians since very ancient times, but not always on the basis of sound science. The first known writings of the use of medicines date back 4000 years or so, to the ancient Egyptians, who used a mixture of minerals and plant-derived concoctions and magic spells to treat disease. Independently, the ancient Indians and Chinese developed their own methods of using of plant- and herb-derived extracts for treating ailments of different kinds, with somewhat variable (and usually not well documented) results. None of these systems for the use of therapeutic substances, collectively often termed 'materia medica', were based on an understanding of the underlying basis of disease (pathology) or of the modes of action of these substances (pharmacology).

In more recent times, our understanding of both pathology and pharmacology, coupled with the use of rigorous clinical trials for the testing of new medicines, has meant that we have a vast and ever-expanding armamentarium of effective medicines available for the treatment of diseases, and for the clinician who is treating patients it is important to understand how they work and why they might often give rise to unwanted side effects.

This is why we have put together this book. Our aim is to give the reader a good understanding of the principles of effective and safe use of medicines in the clinic. We also wish to illustrate how the non-clinical use of pharmacologically active substances, or 'recreational drugs', can present to the clinician.

The most useful way to transmit such knowledge is by the use of real cases, and we hope that the 100 cases we present here will serve this purpose. The first 15 cases cover some important basic principles of clinical pharmacology. The next 75 cases are based on the types of questions that appear in the Prescribing Safety Assessment exam, and will form a good preparation for candidates sitting this exam. The final 10 cases cover other clinically important therapeutic scenarios.

We hope that the reader will find these cases both instructive and interesting.

Kerry Layne and Albert Ferro

AUTHORS

Albert Ferro studied Medicine at King's College London (1978–1984), obtaining a First Class Honours intercalated BSc degree in Biochemistry in 1981 along the way. After qualifying, and following training as a junior doctor in medicine, he completed his PhD in Clinical Pharmacology at Cambridge University. He has been a consultant physician and hypertension specialist at Guy's and St Thomas' Hospitals in London since 1996, and was appointed professor of Clinical Pharmacology at King's College London in 2009. He has published over 150 papers in peer-reviewed journals.

Professor Ferro is ex-vice-president of the British Pharmacological Society (Clinical Section), and previously chaired the Royal College of Physicians Joint Specialty Committee on Clinical Pharmacology & Therapeutics. He served as chair of the London Cardiovascular Society between 2005 and 2009, of which he remains a committee member. He is a fellow of a number of professional societies, including the British Pharmacological Society, British & Irish Hypertension Society, European Society of Cardiology and the Association of Physicians of Great Britain and Ireland. He is editor-in-chief of *JRSM Cardiovascular Disease* and also serves on the editorial boards of several other medical and cardiovascular scientific journals. He currently also chairs the MRCP(UK) Part 1 Board.

Kerry Layne studied medicine at King's College London (2002–2008) and also obtained a First Class Honours intercalated BSc degree in Pharmacology in 2005. She began her junior doctor training at Guy's and St Thomas' NHS Foundation Trust and subsequently specialised in 'General Internal Medicine' and 'Clinical Pharmacology and Therapeutics'. She undertook a PhD in Cardiovascular Medicine during this time. She has recently completed her training and is due to commence a consultant post.

ABBREVIATIONS

ABG	arterial blood gas
ACE	angiotensin converting enzyme
ADP	adenosine diphosphate
ALP	alkaline phosphatase
ALT	alanine aminotransferase
ARB	angiotensin II type 1 receptor blocker
ATP	adenosine triphosphate
BD	twice daily
Bili	bilirubin
BP	blood pressure
Creat	creatinine
CRP	C-reactive protein
CT	computed tomography
DKA	diabetic ketoacidosis
ECG	electrocardiogram
GGT	gamma glutamyl transferase
GTN	glyceryl trinitrate
Hb	haemoglobin
HbA1c	glycated haemoglobin
HCG	human chorionic gonadotropin
HDL	high-density lipoprotein
HIV	human immunodeficiency virus
HR	heart rate
JVP	jugular venous pressure
K	potassium
LDL	low-density lipoprotein
LMWH	low molecular weight heparin
Na	sodium
NIV	non-invasive ventilation
NSAID	non-steroidal anti-inflammatory drug
NT pro-BNP	N-terminal pro-hormone brain natriuretic protein
OD	once daily
Plt	platelet count
QDS	four times daily
RR	respiratory rate
SBP	systolic blood pressure
SpO$_2$	peripheral capillary oxygen saturations
TDS	three times daily
VBG	venous blood gas
VTE	venous thromboembolism
WCC	white cell count

REFERENCE RANGES FOR COMMON INVESTIGATIONS

	Reference range	Units
Full blood count		
White cell count	4.0–11.0	×10⁹/L
Neutrophil count	2.0–7.0	×10⁹/L
Lymphocyte count	1.0–4.0	×10⁹/L
Eosinophil count	0.1–0.4	×10⁹/L
Haemoglobin level	120–160	g/L
Platelet count	150–400	×10⁹/L
Mean corpuscular volume	80–100	fL
Renal profile		
Sodium	135–145	mmol/L
Potassium	3.5–5.0	mmol/L
Urea	2.5–7.8	mmol/L
Creatinine	60–100	µmol/L
Liver function tests		
Bilirubin	05–21	µmol/L
Alanine aminotransferase	05–40	IU/L
Alkaline phosphatase	30–130	IU/L
Gamma glutamyl transferase	7–40	IU/L
Albumin	35–50	g/L
Additional electrolytes		
Corrected calcium	2.20–2.60	mmol/L
Phosphate	0.8–1.3	mmol/L
Magnesium	0.75–1.2	mmol/L
Endocrine tests		
Thyroid stimulating hormone	0.2–5.0	mIU/L
Plasma glucose level	4.0–8.0	mmol/L
HbA1c level	20–42 (4.0–5.9)	mmol/mol (%)
Amylase	<90	IU/L
Inflammatory biomarkers		
C-reactive protein	<1	mg/L
Erythrocyte sedimentation rate	0–22	mm/h
Coagulation tests		
INR	0.8–1.2	
D-dimer	<0.45	µgFEU/mL
Cardiac tests		
NT pro-BNP	<300	ng/L
Troponin T	<14	ng/L

(Continued)

	Reference range	Units
Arterial blood gas		
pH	7.35–7.45	
pO_2	10.5–13.5	kPa
pCO_2	4.7–6.0	kPa
Bicarbonate	22–26	mmol/L
Base excess	–2 to +2	mmol/L
Lactate	0.4–2.0	mmol/L

SECTION 1
BASIC PRINCIPLES

History

A 54-year-old female patient presented to the emergency department with a 6-h history of worsening shortness of breath and sharp, right-sided chest pain that was worse on deep inspiration. She denied experiencing palpitations, did not complain of nausea, and was not feeling lightheaded.

She had a history of recurrent deep vein thromboses for which she was on lifelong warfarin. Her INR had been stable at 3.0–3.5 with 5 mg warfarin once daily for more than a year and had last been checked 4 weeks ago. Her only other past medical history was a recent diagnosis of active pulmonary tuberculosis, for which the patient had been prescribed isoniazid (alongside pyridoxine), rifampicin, pyrazinamide and ethambutol.

The patient worked as a primary school teacher and was usually fit and well. She had never smoked and denied any regular alcohol intake. There was no relevant family history.

Examination

The patient appeared moderately dyspnoeic on exertion but was able to speak comfortably at rest. Her pulse rate was 110 beats per minute and regular and her blood pressure was stable at 130/84 mmHg. Her respiratory rate was 22 breaths per minute. She was afebrile.

Results

Blood test	Result	Reference range
White cell count	7.8×10^9/L	$4.0–11.0 \times 10^9$/L
Haemoglobin	123 g/L	120–160 g/L
Platelet count	400×10^9/L	$150–400 \times 10^9$/L
INR (international normalised ratio)	1.2 units	0.8–1.2 units

A CT pulmonary angiogram scan showed large volume, bilateral pulmonary emboli but no evidence of associated right heart strain.

Questions

1. What is the most likely reason for the patient developing a pulmonary embolus at this point in time?
2. How may this have been prevented?

ANSWERS

1. Although novel oral anti-coagulants are increasingly prescribed for many thrombo-embolic conditions, warfarin remains one of the more commonly prescribed therapies in complex disease.

   The hepatic cytochrome P_{450} (CYP) system consists of a family of isoenzymes that are involved in the metabolism of many drugs, including warfarin. The rate of drug metabolism is affected by a large number of substances, including other medications and dietary sources that can induce or inhibit the activity of the isoenzymes. Table 1.1 shows a selection of substrates that are affected by inducers and inhibitors of the CYP pathways.

   In this instance, the patient has recently commenced treatment with the antibiotic rifampicin, which is a potent inducer of inducer of CYP2C19 – one of the isoenzymes responsible for warfarin metabolism. As the activity of this CYP isoenzyme increases, warfarin is metabolised at a faster rate and may thus reach subtherapeutic levels, which happened in this case and the patient has subsequently developed pulmonary emboli.

2. Warfarin has a narrow therapeutic index, which means that a minor change in dose can cause the drug level to reach sub therapeutic or toxic levels. Warfarin acts by inhibiting vitamin K-dependent synthesis of clotting factors and the INR is used as a measure of the effectiveness of the drug in affecting the prothrombin time.

   In situations where potential CYP inducers or inhibitors are introduced, warfarin therapy must be closely monitored. INR measurements will need to be performed more frequently to allow dose adjustments of warfarin as required, until a point is reached where the patient remains stable on the current therapies. As it can take several days to achieve a therapeutic level of warfarin, an additional agent (typically heparin) will initially need to be prescribed for this patient to ensure that she is adequately anti-coagulated.

Table 1.1 Inducers and inhibitors of cytochrome

Hepatic enzyme inhibition		Hepatic enzyme induction	
Enzyme inhibitors	Drugs with effects potentiated by inhibitors:	Enzyme inducers	Drugs with effects impaired by inducers:
Allopurinol	Carbamazepine	Barbiturates	Hydrocortisone
Cimetidine	Ciclosporin	Carbamazepine	Oral contraceptive pill
Ciprofloxacin	Phenytoin	Ethanol (chronic misuse)	Phenytoin
Disulfiram	Theophyllines	Phenytoin	Warfarin
Erythromycin	Warfarin	Rifampicin	
Ethanol (acute intoxication)		Sulphonylureas	
Isoniazid			
Omeprazole			
Sodium valproate			
Sulphonamides			

🔑	**Key Points**
	1. The CYP system is a family of isoenzymes that are responsible for the metabolism of many drugs.
	2. Enzyme inducers will lead to rapid metabolism of certain drugs and may impair their effects.
	3. Enzyme inhibitors will reduce the rate of metabolism of certain drugs and thus increase their effects.

History

An 85-year-old lady was admitted from a nursing home to the emergency department complaining of worsening shortness of breath and a sensation that her heart was 'racing'. She denied symptoms of chest pain and cough and reported feeling well over recent weeks aside from intermittent episodes of palpitations. Her past medical history included hypertension, ischaemic heart disease and heart failure, as well as a previous episode of atrial fibrillation when she had a community-acquired pneumonia last year. Her regular medications were ramipril 10 mg OD, bendroflumethiazide 2.5 mg OD and digoxin 125 μg OD.

Examination

The patient was afebrile and looked comfortable at rest. Her pulse rate was 140 beats per minute and the blood pressure was 104/70 mmHg. The heart sounds were difficult to hear clearly due to the rapid rate; her pulse was noted to be irregularly irregular. There was mild, pitting oedema to the ankles but her jugular venous pressure was not elevated. Her chest was clear, with oxygen saturations of 97% on room air.

Results

The chest X-ray showed clear lung fields. Her ECG is shown below.

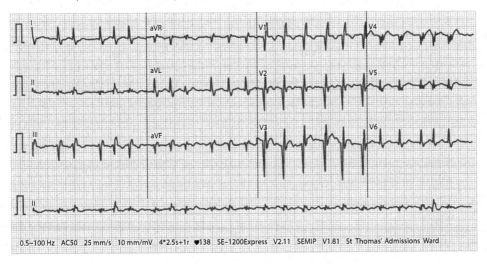

0.5~100 Hz   AC50   25 mm/s   10 mm/mV   4*2.5s+1r   ♥138   SE–1200Express   V2.11   SEMIP   V1.81   St Thomas' Admissions Ward

Questions

1. What would be the next drug of choice for the acute management of this condition?
2. How will you assess whether the patient is on an appropriate dose of digoxin?

ANSWERS

1. The ECG shows atrial fibrillation with a rapid ventricular response and T wave inversions in leads III, VI and V2. Atrial fibrillation is the most common arrhythmia seen in patients over the age of 75 years. Patients who present within 48 h of the onset of atrial fibrillation may be considered for cardioversion therapy to restore sinus rhythm. Beyond this time, the risk of patients developing thrombus formation within the left atrium (and therefore potentially having a stroke) is considered too great and patients should thus be anti-coagulated for at least 3 weeks before being considered for cardioversion therapy.

   In this case, the patient gives a history of having palpitations for weeks and it is uncertain when she developed the arrhythmia. Aside from in cases where the patient is haemodynamically unstable, the first-line strategy in this situation is to achieve rate control by offering either a beta blocker (typically bisoprolol or metoprolol) or a rate-limiting calcium channel blocker (typically diltiazem). Digoxin monotherapy can also be considered for patients who are frail or sedentary, although in this case, the patient is already taking this medication.

2. Digoxin has a narrow therapeutic range and patients taking digoxin may need to have their serum digoxin concentrations measured to ensure that they are not receiving too low a dose, possibly resulting in an inadequate clinical response, or too high a dose and therefore being at risk of digoxin toxicity. Features of digoxin toxicity include arrhythmias (particularly bradycardia or atrioventricular block), abdominal pain, nausea and vomiting, confusion and visual disturbances.

   Digoxin has a long distribution half-life and serum digoxin concentrations should therefore be checked at least 6 h after the patient receives the dose. Levels should be checked routinely in patients who have started digoxin within the past 2 weeks, patients with renal impairment, and in patients at increased risk of toxicity, such as those taking drugs that may interact or who have hypokalaemia. It is important to remember that there is an overlap between therapeutic and toxic levels, and you should therefore consider a diagnosis of digoxin toxicity in patients who have the appropriate clinical signs and symptoms, even if their serum digoxin level is within the therapeutic range.

 Key Points

1. Patients who are experiencing atrial fibrillation with a rapid ventricular response rate can be given various pharmacological therapies to slow down their heart rate, including beta blockers, calcium channel blockers and digoxin.
2. Digoxin has a narrow therapeutic range and patients taking digoxin may need to have their serum digoxin concentrations measured to ensure that they are not receiving doses that are too high or too low.

History

A 40-year-old man presented to hospital complaining of vomiting. He described a 2-day history of abdominal pain associated with vomiting and diarrhoea. He denied experiencing fevers, cough or urinary tract symptoms. He had no unwell contacts and had not travelled abroad in the past year. His past medical history included bipolar affective disorder, for which he took a total of 1200 mg lithium daily in divided doses. This dose had recently been increased by the community mental health team due to recurrent episodes of mania.

Examination

The patient was afebrile and appeared comfortable at rest. His mucus membranes appeared dry. His heart rate was 95 beats per minute and his blood pressure was 100/64 mmHg. His abdomen was mildly tender throughout but soft with normal bowel sounds. He was noted to have a resting tremor affecting both hands.

Results

Bloods: WCC 4.6, Hb 128, Plt 211, Na 134, K 3.5, Creat 84, CRP 2

Lithium level 2.5 (reference range 0.6–1.2 mEq/L)

Questions

1. What is the most likely cause of the patient's symptoms?
2. How will you treat this patient?

ANSWERS

1. The patient presents with a 2-day history of abdominal pain, vomiting and diarrhoea. He shows signs of dehydration (dry mucus membranes plus mild tachycardia and hypotension) and also reportedly has a resting tremor. These signs are consistent with lithium toxicity, which is confirmed by his blood results that show elevated lithium levels.

   Lithium has a narrow therapeutic window, which means that toxicity can develop with minor changes in dose or drug excretion. In this case, the patient reports a recent increase in his dose. Lithium levels are typically closely monitored, particularly if dose adjustments have been made.

2. Lithium is rapidly absorbed and does not undergo metabolism. It is primarily renally excreted with around 80% of the drug being reabsorbed in the proximal convoluted tubule. When patients are dehydrated or hyponatraemic, there is greater lithium reabsorption and thus higher circulating concentrations.

   In this case, it is unclear whether the diarrhoea and vomiting are symptoms of the lithium toxicity, or whether a pre-existing episode of gastroenteritis has led to sodium and fluid losses that have then prompted greater reabsorption of lithium. It is also worth noting that long-term treatment with lithium can result in nephrogenic diabetes insipidus due to interference with anti-diuretic hormone activity.

   This patient will need intravenous fluid rehydration with careful monitoring of her sodium levels. Her fluid status should be regularly assessed. In cases of severe lithium toxicity, haemodialysis can be commenced as a form of renal replacement therapy to increase lithium excretion.

 Key Points

1. Lithium has a narrow therapeutic window and patients can develop signs of toxicity with minor dose adjustments.
2. Lithium is primarily renally excreted. In cases of overdose with severe toxicity, haemodialysis may need to be commenced to increase excretion of lithium.

CASE 4: DRUG INTERACTIONS

History

A 24-year-old woman presented to the hospital with lower abdominal pain and vomiting. She reported that the symptoms had developed suddenly, approximately 45-min earlier. She had felt well earlier in the day and denied any other symptoms. She had eaten some toast for breakfast and nothing since. She had not experienced any diarrhoea and had no contacts with similar symptoms. Her past medical history included gastro-oesophageal reflux disease and a recent diagnosis of pulmonary tuberculosis, for which she was being treated currently. Her regular medications included: isoniazid, rifampin, pyrazinamide, omeprazole and the combined oral contraceptive pill. She worked as a salesperson and did not smoke, drink alcohol or take recreational drugs.

Examination

The patient appeared pale and distressed. Her heart rate was 140 bpm and her blood pressure was 106/74 mmHg. Her abdomen was generally tender, with particularly pain over the right iliac fossa, with guarding present.

Results

Bloods: WCC 14.2, Hb 105, Plt 460, Na 135, K 3.8, Creat 60, CRP 122

Urine dip: positive for leucocytes, and positive for the beta subunit of human chorionic gonadotropin (hCG)

Questions

1. What diagnoses should be considered for this young woman presenting with sudden-onset right iliac fossa pain?
2. Are there any potential interactions from her medication history that should be considered?

ANSWERS

1. There is a broad differential diagnosis for right iliac fossa pain. Assuming the patient has no past history of appendicectomy, appendicitis is one of the likely diagnoses and an urgent ultrasound or CT scan of the patient's abdomen should be arranged to look for signs of this.

   Pyelonephritis is a common cause of abdominal pain and vomiting and occurs more frequently in female patients. This patient's blood tests show elevated inflammatory markers and her urine dip is positive for leucoyctes, which may indicate a urinary tract infection. The patient has not reported dysuria or fevers, however, and pain from pyelonephritis typically has a gradual onset, rather than a sudden onset as with this case. Renal colic is another possibility, although patients typically complain of pain radiating from the flank to the groin, which comes on in spasms. The presence of renal stones usually results in red blood cells being detected on the urine dipstick test also.

   The patient has a positive pregnancy test (hCG present on the urine dip) and thus the most important diagnosis to exclude is an ectopic pregnancy, where the fertilised egg has implanted outside the uterus, usually in the fallopian tube. As the ectopic pregnancy progresses, the fallopian tube can rupture requiring emergency surgery.

2. The patient is taking the oral contraceptive pill, which has a 9% annual pregnancy rate with typical use, and less than 1% annual pregnancy rate with correct use. The effectiveness of both the combined (contains an oestrogen and a progesterone) and the progesterone-only oral contraceptive pill, as well as the etonogestrel-releasing contraceptive implant, are considerably reduced by co-administration of drugs that induce hepatic enzyme activity.

   Such medications promote upregulation of the hepatic cytochrome P_{450} system, thus increasing the rate of metabolism of other drugs that are metabolised by cytochrome P_{450}, including most hormonal oral contraceptives.

   This case highlights the importance of reviewing potential drug interactions whenever a new medication is commenced, and considering methods to reduce the impact of this. In this situation, the patient needed treatment for pulmonary tuberculosis with the enzyme-inducing drug, rifampicin, and should thus have been advised to consider alternative methods of contraception, such as condom use or intra-uterine device insertion, to reduce the chance of pregnancy. You should ideally take the opportunity to review a patient's drug history at every new clinical encounter and consider potential interactions between their medications. As the use of electronic prescribing increases, prescribers are now often automatically alerted to potential drug interactions when they prescribe a medication, thus reducing the risk of harm to patients.

 Key Points

1. The efficacy of many oral contraceptive agents is reduced by co-administration of drugs that induce hepatic enzyme activity.
2. As a prescriber, you should review potential drug interactions whenever a new medication is commenced, and consider methods to reduce the impact of this.

CASE 5: MONOCLONAL ANTIBODY THERAPY

History

A 32-year-old woman was attending the rheumatology clinic for review of her rheumatoid arthritis. For the past 3 years, her rheumatoid arthritis had been poorly controlled. She had experienced painful swelling of her hands and feet, and joint stiffness that lasted for 60–90 min each morning. She also felt fatigued and had noticed some unintentional weight loss. She had no other past medical history. Her regular medications included prednisolone 10 mg OD and omeprazole 20mg OD. She had trialled courses of naproxen, methotrexate, sulfasalazine and hydroxychloroquine over the past 2 years, with no significant improvement in her symptoms. She had no known drug allergies. She worked as a journalist, drank 5–10 units of alcohol per week and had never smoked.

Examination

The patient appeared comfortable at rest and was afebrile. The wrists in additional to the small joints of the hands and feet were swollen bilaterally; the joints were warm to touch. There was reduced range of movement when attempting to make a fist with the left hand and when extending both wrists. The large joints appeared to be unaffected.

Results

Bloods: WCC 11.6 (neutrophils 7.8), Hb 106, MCV 80, Plt 260, CRP 47, ESR 69

Questions

1. The patient has trialled multiple treatment courses over the past 2 years without significant improvement of her rheumatoid arthritis symptoms. What is the next class of medication that should be trialled?
2. What are the potential adverse effects associated with this class of medication?

ANSWERS

1. The patient has trialled courses of non-steroidal anti-inflammatory drugs (NSAIDs), steroids, and at least 2 disease-modifying anti-rheumatic drugs (DMARDs; methotrexate and hydroxychloroquine). The next step would be to commence a biologic agent – these are typically administered either subcutaneously or intravenously and are used in combination with a non-biologic DMARD.

   The disease process in rheumatoid arthritis is primarily mediated by pro-inflammatory cytokines, including interleukin-1 (IL-1) and tumour necrosis factor-alpha (TNF-α), and biologic agents act to modify these inflammatory pathways. Examples of these drugs, include:

   a. TNF-inhibitors, such as the circulating receptor fusion protein, etanercept, or the monoclonal antibodies, adalimumab and infliximab.
   b. The IL-1 receptor antagonist protein, anakinra.
   c. The B-cell target drug, rituximab. This drug is a monoclonal antibody against CD20, which is a B-lymphocyte antigen that is found on the surface of B-cells.
   d. The T-cell target drug, abatacept. T-cells are activated when the CD28 antigen on the T-cell binds to the CD80 and CD86 molecules on antigen presenting cells. Abatacept is a fusion protein that binds to CD80 and CD86 molecules to competitively inhibit this reaction.

2. Some patients develop infusion reactions whilst receiving biologic therapies. These can either be localised (pain and erythema around the injection site) or systemic (flushing, nausea, tachycardia, or anaphylaxis). Intravenous biologic therapies are thus administered in controlled environments where specialist nurses or doctors are available to monitor observations and provide treatment with antihistamines and anti-emetics as required.

   As biologic therapies suppress the function of the immune system, patients are more prone to developing infections, including serious infections, such as pneumonia, that require hospital admission. Patients receiving biologic therapies, particularly anti-TNF drugs, are at risk of reactivation of latent tuberculosis infections.

   In rare cases, rituximab therapy has been associated with the development of the demyelimating disease, progressive multifocal leukoencephalopathy (PML).

 Key Points

1. Biologic agents, such as TNF-inhibitors, may be commenced in patients with rheumatoid arthritis who have not responded sufficiently to NSAIDs, steroids and DMARDs.
2. Patients who commence biologic therapies should be advised that they are at increased risk of developing infections due to suppression of their immune system.

CASE 6: LIGAND-GATED ION CHANNELS

History
A 24-year-old woman presented to the emergency department complaining of a 2-week history of blurred vision. Her symptoms had come on gradually, and had become progressively worse. She reported that the blurred vision was particularly prominent when she was watching the television at night. She had no other past medical history and took no regular medications. There was no significant family history. The patient worked as a lifeguard in a local leisure centre. She had never smoked, did not use any recreational drugs and consumed approximately 10 units of alcohol per week.

Examination
The patient was alert and orientated. Her cardiovascular, respiratory and abdominal systems showed no abnormal findings. Neurological examination identified bilateral ptosis, which worsened on sustained upward gaze.

Results
Chest X-ray: A left hilar mass, approximately 20 mm × 15 mm (see black arrow)

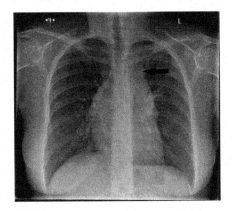

Questions
1. Describe the pathophysiology of the likely underlying condition.
2. What medication options are available to treat the patient?

ANSWERS

1. The patient has presented with intermittent blurring of vision and a bilateral ptosis that worsens on sustained upwards gaze. These findings are typical for myasthenia gravis, an autoimmune condition that is characterised by fatigable muscle weakness. Patients typically present with eye signs, including blurring of vision that occurs due to weakness of the extraocular muscles, but symptoms can progress to involve multiple muscle groups, including the bulbar and proximal limb muscles.

   Myasthenia gravis is an acquired disease where autoantibodies develop against the post-synaptic nicotinic acetylcholine receptor, or a protein called 'muscle-specific kinase' (MuSK). Typically, when acetylcholine is released from the synaptic vesicles in the pre-synaptic nerve terminal into the synaptic cleft, it diffuses across the synaptic cleft and binds to the acetylcholine receptors on the postsynaptic muscle membrane, resulting in depolarisation of the muscle membrane and the subsequent generation of an action potential (see Figure 6.1a). Acetylcholinesterase enzymes break down acetylcholine in the synaptic cleft, thus terminating the action potential. In myasthenia gravis, autoantibody destruction results in fewer acetylcholine receptors and thus there are reduced action potentials generated and muscles are thus weaker (see Figure 6.1b).

   Approximately 10%–15% of patients with myasthenia gravis have a thymoma, which is a tumour originating from the epithelial cells of the thymus – in this case, the patient's chest x-ray shows a left hilar mass, which may represent a thymoma.

2. Acetylcholinesterase inhibitors, such as pyridostigmine and neostigmine, reduce the breakdown of acetylcholine in the synaptic cleft, therefore enabling greater binding to the acetylcholine receptors, improving action potential generation.

   Patients with a thymoma may benefit from surgical thymectomy, and in severe cases of myasthenia gravis, plasmapheresis (to remove the autoantibodies) and intravenous immunoglobulin (to bind the autoantibodies) may also be considered.

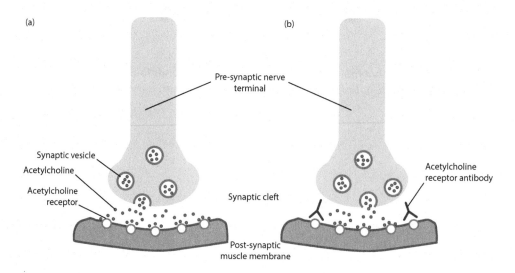

Figure 6.1 The neuromuscular junction in healthy individuals (a) and in individuals with myasthenia gravis (b).

🔑	Key Points

1. Myasthenia gravis develops when patients form autoantibodies against the post-synaptic nicotinic acetylcholine receptor, or the MuSK protein.
2. Acetylcholinesterase inhibitors increase the quantities of acetylcholine in the synaptic cleft, thus improving symptoms of weakness.

CASE 7: ACETYLATION

History

A 43-year-old man presents to hospital complaining of a 24-h history of jaundice and abdominal pain. He has been feeling generally unwell for the past week and his appetite has been reduced. His past medical history includes pulmonary tuberculosis, for which he is currently being treated with isoniazid, rifampin and pyrazinamide. He works as an office manager, does not drink alcohol, takes no recreational drugs and has never smoked.

Examination

The patient is visibly jaundiced. His heart sounds are normal and his chest is clear. His abdomen is soft throughout, with marked right upper quadrant tenderness. His bowel sounds were normal. There were no visibly stigmata of chronic liver disease. His calves were soft and non-tender with no peripheral oedema.

Results

Bloods: Bilirubin 78, ALT 350, ALP 190, Albumin 38, INR 1.2

Questions

1. The patient is subsequently diagnosed with likely drug-induced hepatotoxicity, and the on-call medical consultant suggests that either rifampicin or isoniazid could be responsible. Name some of the potential factors that may make people more prone to drug-induced hepatotoxicity.
2. How would this patient's 'acetylator status' affect their risk of drug-induced hepatotoxicity?

ANSWERS

1. In general, patients are more likely to develop hepatotoxicity if they have any under-lying liver conditions, including hepatitis, hepatic malignancy and cirrhotic liver disease. Risk factors include: increasing age, malnutrition, chronic alcoholism, HIV infection, and the concomitant administration of other hepatotoxic drugs.
2. This patient is taking isoniazid, which is primarily metabolised by acetylation by liver N-acetyltransferase to acetyl-isoniazid. Acetylation occurs when an acetyl functional group is introduced into a chemical compound. There are two genotypic variants in N-acetylation, and patients may be 'rapid acetylators' or 'slow acetyl-ators' depending on which variant they have inherited. The half-life of isoniazid thus has two peaks (a bimodal distribution), at 1 h and 3 h.

   Approximately 50% of Caucasian and Afro-Caribbean people are rapid acetyl-ators, whereas the majority of Asian people are rapid acetylators. Slow acetylation can result in higher concentrations of toxic metabolites of drugs, and thus increase the risk of adverse events occurring following drug administration. Other drugs that are metabolised by acetylation include dapsone, hydralazine, procainamide and sulfamethazine.

 Key Points

1. Patients with underlying risk factors, such as malnutrition, HIV infection and chronic alcoholism are more susceptible to drug-induced hepatotoxicity.
2. Patients may be 'rapid acetylators' or 'slow acetylators'. Slow acetylation can result in higher concentrations of toxic metabolites of drugs, increasing the risk of occur-rence of adverse drug events.

History

A 68-year-old man came to hospital complaining of chest pain that had developed whilst he was running for a bus. The pain was crushing in nature and was located in the centre of his chest, radiating to his left arm and jaw. He reported using his 'red spray' and the pain subsequently resolved. His past medical history included angina, hypertension and hypercholesterolaemia. His regular medications were amlodipine 10 mg OD, ramipril 10 mg OD and atorvastatin 40 mg ON. He was an ex-smoker with a 20-pack year history and drank 25 units of alcohol per week. He was a retired security officer and lived with his wife and grandchild.

Examination

Systems examination was unremarkable.

Results

ECG: normal sinus rhythm, Troponin T – 11

Questions

1. The 'red spray' that the patient used was glyceryl trinitrate (GTN). What is the mechanism of action for this drug?
2. Why is the sublingual formulation of GTN favoured in acute angina?

ANSWERS

1. GTN is a 'nitric oxide donor' drug that is commonly prescribed to treat symptoms of ischaemic heart disease. Metabolism of GTN results in increased generation of nitric oxide, which is a potent vasodilator. Nitric oxide increases cellular concentrations of cyclic guanosine monophosphate (cGMP), which subsequently initiates relaxation of vascular smooth muscle cells. This promotes dilatation of the venous and arterial systems and both the pre-load and after-load are thus reduced. Coronary artery dilatation will additionally improve the delivery of oxygenated blood to the heart during episodes of angina.

2. GTN is available in a variety of forms and is rapidly absorbed sublingually or via the gastrointestinal tract. When taken orally, GTN undergoes extensive hepatic first-pass metabolism, which greatly reduces its bioavailability. Sublingual GTN is therefore preferable in acute events, as this provides a more potent effect. Sublingual GTN can be delivered via either a spray or tablets; the tablets expire within 8 weeks of opening the packet, however, and thus the spray is generally preferred. Peak drug levels are achieved within 2 min of administration of sublingual GTN.

   GTN can be delivered via an intravenous infusion in a hospital setting – this allows medical staff to accurately titrate the dose to manage the balance of reducing pre-load and after-load, whilst maintaining an adequate perfusing blood pressure. GTN patches are also available, to provide a continuous background dose transdermally. This is typically a low dose of GTN and is typically used in patients with hypertension who are unable to tolerate oral medications.

   Of note, tolerance to GTN develops rapidly when it is used continually over a number of hours, potentially due to the development of intracellular oxidative stress and endothelial dysfunction. GTN patches may, therefore, need to be removed overnight for 8 h to restore the patient's physiological response to GTN, and similarly, infusions of GTN may need to be intermittently stopped. Some studies suggest that up to 50% of Asian people possess an inactive mutant form of a gene that produces an enzyme involved in the production of nitric oxide in response to GTN and the drug may therefore be less effective in this population.

 Key Points

1. GTN is a 'nitric oxide donor' that increases dilation of both venous and arterial blood vessels.
2. Tolerance to GTN can develop following ongoing exposure over a number of hours and it thus becomes less effective over time when administered via a continuous infusion or topically via a patch.

History

A 72-year-old man attends the emergency department following a fall. He reports that whilst walking from the living room to the kitchen, he tripped on the corner of the rug and fell forwards onto his knees. He denies sustaining any head injury but does complain of pain over his left wrist. This is his third hospital attendance with a fall in the past month. He has no significant past medical history and takes no regular medications. The patient is a retired painter and decorator, he lives alone and has no package of care. He does not drink alcohol regularly and is an ex-smoker with a 30-pack year history.

Examination

The patient is alert and orientated to time, place and person. He has no visible injuries. Cardiovascular, respiratory and abdominal system examinations are unremarkable. Neurological examination identifies bilateral increased tone in the upper limbs with a pronounced resting tremor, consistent with 'cogwheel rigidity'. There is a slow, rhythmic 'pill-rolling' tremor in the left hand. The patient's face appears expressionless, or 'mask-like' and his speech is monotonous. He walks with a shuffling gait.

Questions

1. This patient is likely to have an underlying diagnosis of Parkinson's disease. Why should you prescribe levodopa, rather than dopamine, to this patient?
2. Are there any additional medications that can be prescribed to enhance the efficacy of levodopa?

ANSWERS

1. Movement control is governed by multiple, complex neural pathways working in tandem. One such pathway involves neurons located within the substantia nigra, in the ventral midbrain that communicate with the basal ganglia via the neurotransmitter, dopamine. Parkinson's disease develops when there is degeneration of dopamine-producing cells in the substantia nigra, resulting in reduced levels of dopamine available for neurotransmission.

   Exogenous dopamine can be administered to patients, however dopamine is water-soluble and hydrophilic and thus unable to cross the blood–brain barrier. Levodopa, a dopamine pro-drug, is able to cross the blood–brain barrier via an amino acid transport system, where it is then converted to dopamine.

2. When administered orally, levodopa is absorbed by the gastrointestinal tract and converted to dopamine by a dopa decarboxylase (DDC) inhibitor. To prevent conversion to dopamine occurring in the periphery (thus requiring larger doses to be administered and inducing greater adverse effects), levodopa is combined with a peripheral dopa decarboxylase inhibitor, such as carbidopa. Peripheral DDC inhibitors are unable to cross the blood–brain barrier, enabling levodopa to be transported to the brain, where it is then converted to dopamine.

   Levodopa is also metabolised to 3-O-MDopa by the catechol-O-methyltransferase (COMT) enzyme. COMT inhibitors, such as tolcapone and entacapone, can reduce the peripheral breakdown of levodopa (Figure 9.1).

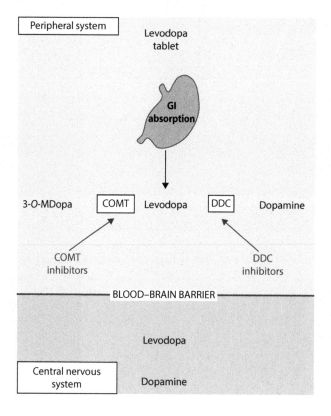

Figure 9.1 Levodopa pharmacokinetics.

🔑	Key Points

1. Dopamine is unable to cross the blood–brain barrier, whilst levodopa, a dopamine pro-drug, is able to cross the blood–brain barrier via an amino acid transport system, where it is then converted to dopamine.
2. Levodopa is typically combined with a peripheral dopa decarboxylase inhibitor to ensure maximal doses reach the central nervous system.

CASE 10: ABSORPTION

History

A 75-year-old woman was admitted to hospital following a fall at home. She tripped over an object on the floor and fell onto her right side. The patient's carer was with her at the time and helped her back to her feet whilst waiting for the ambulance to arrive. The patient reported feeling well aside from pain over her right arm. Her past medical history included multiple previous falls, which had resulted in fractures to the left wrist and the left hip. She additionally reported postural hypotension and recurrent urinary tract infections. Her regular medications included a combination tablet of calcium carbonate and vitamin D_3 1500 mg/400 IU twice daily, and paracetamol 1 g QDS. She lived alone with a twice daily package of care to assist with meal preparation. She did not drink alcohol and had never smoked.

Examination

The patient had extensive bruising over the right upper arm and a laceration to the forehead. Systems examination was unremarkable. The patient reported difficulty moving her shoulder and elbow joints in all planes due to pain.

Results

An X-ray of the right upper limb showed that the patient's right humerus was fractured.

A DEXA scan was compatible with osteoporosis.

Questions

1. This patient was informed that she has been diagnosed with osteoporosis, which likely contributed to her previous fractures. She was advised to take alendronic acid 70 mg once weekly to treat her osteoporosis. What is the mechanism of action of alendronic acid?
2. The patient's carer will be administering the new medication. They have asked whether there are any particular instructions that the patient should follow when taking alendronic acid – what should you advise them?

ANSWERS

1. Alendronic acid (or alendronate) is a bisphosphonate that acts to reduce bone loss by inhibiting osteoclastic bone resorption. Alendronic acid, as with other bisphosphonates, has a very high affinity for bone mineral relative to other tissues, and thus deposits throughout the skeleton.

2. Alendronic acid, as with other oral bisphosphonates, is associated with the development of multiple upper-gastrointestinal adverse effects, including erosive oesophagitis. For this reason, it is advised that patients take the tablet with a full glass of water and that they remain sitting upright or standing for 30–60 min following this. Patients should particularly be advised to avoid bending down/leaning forwards or retaining the tablets in their mouth (e.g. sucking them), which can cause local irritation.

   Alendronic acid has an extremely low oral bioavailability of around 0.6%–1.0% compared to a reference intravenous dose in the fasted state, which is in keeping with other oral bisphosphonate preparations. Alendronic acid is polar at physiological pH, binding to available cations with high affinity, and absorption of alendronic acid is negligible in the presence of food. Patients are thus advised to take the dose of alendronic acid at least 30 min before their first food or drink of the day, with a glass of tap (not mineral) water.

 Key Points

1. Alendronic acid has a high affinity for bone tissue and deposits throughout the skeleton.
2. Alendronic acid has a low oral bioavailability and patients are thus encouraged to maximise absorption by avoiding food and drink prior to taking the drug.

History

A 50-year-old Caucasian man attends his general practitioner for a review of his blood pressure control. He was found to be hypertensive at a routine physical assessment 6 months earlier and had since been attempting to improve his diet and increase the amount of exercise that he regularly undertook. He has been feeling well, with no recent illnesses. His past medical history includes gastro-oesophageal reflux disease, chronic lower back pain and hypercholesterolaemia. His regular medications are omeprazole 40 mg OD and simvastatin 20 mg ON. The patient works as a barrister, smokes 20 cigarettes daily and drinks 20–30 units of alcohol per week.

Examination

The patient is overweight with a BMI of 27.2. His heart rate is 82 bpm and his blood pressure is 158/92 mmHg. Systems examination is otherwise unremarkable.

Results

Bloods: Na 140, K 3.7, Creat 70, HbA1c level 5.8% (consistent with non-diabetes)

24-h ambulatory blood pressure monitoring:

- Average 24-h blood pressure 160/94 mmHg
- Average daytime blood pressure 170/98 mmHg
- Average night-time blood pressure 150/86 mmHg

Questions

1. The patient's general practitioner diagnoses hypertension and recommends that the patient commence ramipril. What is the mechanism of action of this drug?
2. Other that ACE-inhibitors, can you describe any other pharmacological therapies that target the renin-angiotensin-aldosterone axis?

ANSWERS

1. Ramipril is an angiotensin-converting enzyme (ACE) inhibitor. Other examples of ACE inhibitors include enalapril, lisinopril and perindopril.

   The renin-angiotensin-aldosterone axis is part of the body's homeostatic mechanisms to regulate the blood pressure, ensuring adequate organ perfusion. In response to a reduction in blood pressure, the enzyme renin, is secreted by the renal juxtaglomerular cells. Renin cleaves angiotensinogen, an α-2-globulin produced by the liver into the peptide hormone, angiotensin I. Angiotensin I does not appear to have significant physiological effects, but it is subsequently cleaved by the ACE into angiotensin II.

   Angiotensin II acts on angiotensin type 1 receptors to induce vasoconstriction and also stimulates increased production of vasopressin (anti-diuretic hormone), therefore increasing the blood pressure. Angiotensin II additionally induces increased secretion of the mineralocorticoid hormone, aldosterone, which acts to promote sodium and water retention, thus further increasing the blood pressure; see Figure 11.1. In addition to a reduction in mean arterial pressure, ACE inhibitors can reduce left ventricular remodelling following myocardial infarction.

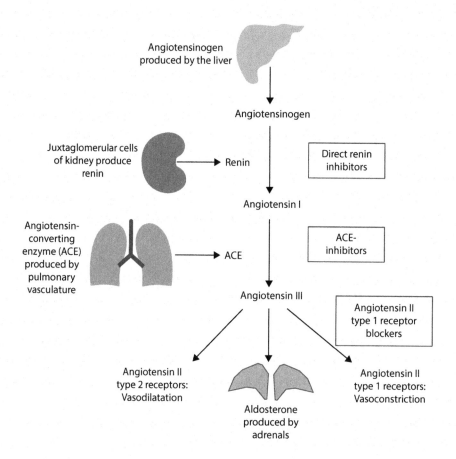

Figure 11.1 The renin-angiotensin-aldosterone axis.

2. ACE inhibitors are commonly used therapies in the management of hypertension and heart failure but can be poorly tolerated by some patients. In addition to its role in the renin-angiotensin-aldosterone axis, ACE also breaks down the peptide, bradykinin, into inactive metabolites. Bradykinin is an inflammatory mediator, and reduced breakdown of bradykinin can result in bronchoconstriction (resulting in a dry cough), or angioedema in some cases.

Additional pharmacological targets in the renin-angiotensin-aldosterone axis include renin, and the direct renin inhibitor, aliskiren, may be used in some cases to antagonise renin and reduce the production of angiotensin I.

More commonly, the angiotensin II type 1 receptor is targeted by drugs, such as losartan and valsartan, that competitively antagonise these receptors. Angiotensin II type 1 receptor blockers (ARBs) reduce vasoconstriction and thus reduce the mean arterial pressure. They also leave the angiotensin II type 2 receptor unopposed, which may additionally promote vasodilatation.

 | **Key Points**
---

1. The renin-angiotensin-aldosterone axis is part of the body's homeostatic mechanisms to regulate the blood pressure.
2. There are multiple therapeutic targets for the renin-angiotensin-aldosterone. Drugs that target this system include ACE-inhibitors, ARBs and, in some cases, direct renin-inhibitors.

History

A 72-year-old man developed central crushing chest pain whilst rushing to catch a train. The pain radiated to his left arm and up to his jaw. He complained of associated nausea and shortness of breath. He had not experienced similar episodes in the past. His past medical history included hypertension and prostate benign prostatic hyperplasia. His regular medications were amlodipine 10 mg OD and ramipril 2.5 mg OD. He was a retired optician, did not smoke and was independent for all activities of daily living.

Examination

The patient's blood pressure was 146/94 mmHg. His heart rate was 90 bpm. His heart sounds were normal and his chest was clear. The jugular venous pressure was not elevated and there was no peripheral oedema.

Results

The patient's ECG showed ST-segment elevation in leads II, III and aVF, in keeping with an inferior myocardial infarction.

Questions

1. The patient was given 300 mg of aspirin by the paramedics prior to arriving to hospital. How does aspirin exert its anti-platelet effects?
2. Aspirin can increase the risk of gastrointestinal bleeding. Discuss the mechanism(s) that lead to this adverse effect.

ANSWERS

1. The primary function of platelets is to prevent haemorrhage. Circulating platelets move from a resting state to an activated state in response to signs of damage to the vascular endothelium. Activated platelets adhere to the endothelium, aggregating to form a haemostatic plug that reduces bleeding.

   At sites of atherosclerotic disease, plaque rupture leads to activation and aggregation of platelets and subsequent atherothrombotic disease, which can result in ischaemic injuries, including myocardial infarction and stroke. In order to reduce the risk of such events, patients who have signs of atherothrombotic disease, or those are considered to be high risk of developing this, are prescribed anti-platelet therapy, such as aspirin.

   Aspirin, otherwise known as salicylic acid, irreversibly binds to and inhibits the cyclo-oxygenase (COX) enzymes. The cyclo-oxygenase enzymes convert arachidonic acid into prostaglandin H_2. Prostaglandin H_2 is subsequently converted by tissue-specific synthases into the eicosanoids, thromboxane A_2, prostacyclin and prostaglandin. These eicosanoids play complex roles in inflammation and platelet homeostasis. By inhibiting the COX enzymes, aspirin reduces both platelet activation and aggregation, thus reducing the risk of thromboembolic disease; Figure 12.1.

2. As well as functioning as an anti-platelet drug, aspirin is additionally classed as a non-steroidal anti-inflammatory drug (NSAID). NSAIDs inhibit the COX enzymes, thus reducing gastric prostaglandin synthesis. Gastric prostaglandins are a key component in gastric mucosal defence – they inhibit acid secretion, stimulate bicarbonate and mucus production, and increase gastric mucosal flow. By inhibiting these actions, aspirin and other NSAIDs promote damage to the gastric mucosa, thus increasing the risk of upper gastrointestinal bleeding events.

   Additionally, as mentioned in answer 1, aspirin inhibits the COX enzymes and thus modifies platelet homestostatic mechanisms to disrupt platelet activation and aggregation. This results in impaired clot formation and a prolonged bleeding time.

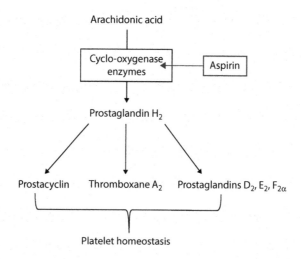

Figure 12.1 Inhibition of cyclo-oxygenase enzymes by aspirin.

🔑	**Key Points**
	1. Aspirin irreversibly binds to and inhibits the COX enzymes to reduce platelet activation and aggregation.
	2. Aspirin increases the risk of gastrointestinal bleeding by reducing gastric prostaglandin synthesis, thus promoting damage to the gastric mucosa.

History

A 21-year-old woman presented to her general practitioner complaining of a throbbing pain over the right side of her head. The onset of the headache was preceded by an awareness of 'flashing lights' in the patient's vision. The pain was worsened by movement and bright lights and was relieved by resting in a dark, quiet room. There was associated nausea; she had vomited several times. She had experienced 5–6 similar episodes over the past year with no clear trigger. Each episode lasted for approximately 12–18 h and resolved spontaneously. The patient had no significant past medical history and had been well over recent weeks. She took no regular medications but did have an intrauterine system *in situ*. The patient worked as an engineering apprentice and she had not travelled abroad in the past year.

Examination

The patient was afebrile. Her heart rate was 94 bpm and her blood pressure was 110/70 mmHg. Neurological examination was unremarkable. The patient was not objectively photophobic, there was no nuchal rigidity and Kernig's sign was not positive.

Results

Bloods: WCC 5.6, Hb 114, MCV 80, Plt 401, Na 140, K 4.0, Creat 60, CRP <1

Urine dip: negative for blood, leucocytes, nitrites, protein and glucose. β-HCG negative

Questions

1. Which medications would you consider prescribing to treat this patient's headache?
2. Describe the mechanism of action for triptan analgesia.

ANSWERS

1. This patient is likely to be experiencing migraines. Although the pathophysiology underlying the condition is not fully established, it is thought that migraine sufferers are prone to entering a state of 'altered excitability of the brain'. This may occur due to a complex series of neurogenic and vascular events within the central nervous system, including abnormal activation of the trigeminovascular pathways.

   Those who experience migraines present with a multitude of symptoms, but classical features of migraine include a severe, pulsatile or throbbing, unilateral headache that develops over hours and may last for 24–48 h. Photophobia and phonophobia are common features and the headache is typically worse on moving. Patients typically experience nausea and they may vomit. A variety of neurological features may also transiently develop, including paraesthesia, hemiparesis and aphasia.

   Patients often find that simple analgesics, including non-steroidal anti-inflammatory drugs (NSAIDs) and paracetamol are effective at reducing the pain associated with the migraine or terminating it altogether, particularly if they are used within 15 min of symptom onset. Stronger analgesics, for example, codeine phosphate, may be beneficial in some patients, although opioids may worsen symptoms of nausea and frequent use of these agents may result in dependence.

   The dopamine D_2 antagonist, metoclopramide, has been commonly used to treat nausea and gastric stasis and to improve the gastrointestinal absorption of analgesics in migraine. Studies suggest that the H_1 and D_2 antagonist, promethazine and parenteral metoclopramide may also relieve migrainous headaches without the addition of analgesics, although adverse effects associated with both single and repeated uses of these drugs include acute transient dystonic reactions and tardive dyskinesia.

   Triptans and ergot alkaloids are commonly used to terminate migrainous headaches and these are discussed below.

2. Triptans, such as sumatriptan and zolmitriptan, are 5-hydroxytryptamine (5-HT) receptor agonists, with particular selectivity for the 5-HT_{1B} and 5-HT_{1D} receptors, which are located on vascular smooth muscle cells, and perivascular trigeminal nerve terminals respectively. 5-HT_{1B} agonism results in intracranial extracerebral vasoconstriction, which eases pain from migraionous headaches, and 5-HT_{1D} agonism inhibits the release of pro-inflammatory neuropeptides that may convey nociceptive information to the thalamus. Triptan administration can result in vasoconstriction of the coronary arteries and thus must be used with caution in patients with potential coronary artery atheromatous disease.

   Ergot alkaloids, such as ergotamine, are agonists of the α-adrenoceptors, 5-HT receptors, and dopamine D_2 receptors. The mechanism of action of ergot alkaloids is not entirely understood, although, similarly to triptans, their therapeutic effects are likely to be produced via agonism of the 5-HT_{1B} and 5-HT_{1D} receptors to promote vasoconstriction of the intracranial blood vessels and to inhibit trigeminal neurotransmission.

🔑	Key Points
	1. There are a variety of drugs that may be used to treat migraine headaches, including simple analgesics, opioid analgesics, dopamine D_2 antagonists, triptans and ergot alkaloids.
	2. Triptans are commonly used to terminate migrainous headaches, and these act via agonism of the 5-HT$_{1B}$ and 5-HT$_{1D}$ receptors to promote vasoconstriction of the intracranial blood vessels and to inhibit trigeminal neurotransmission.

History and examination

A 40-year-old man was brought to hospital after being found collapsed in the street. He had a syringe and needle in his hand when he was found. The paramedics examined the patient and found that he was unresponsive to voice and pain. His pupils were 1–2 mm bilaterally. His heart rate was 50 bpm and his respiratory rate was 4 breaths per minute. No other positive findings were elicited on systemic examination.

The paramedics diagnosed opioid toxicity and administered naloxone. The patient regained consciousness and was brought to hospital where he recovered well. His blood results were sent for toxicological screening and were positive for both fentanyl and heroin. The patient expressed an ongoing desire to abstain from intravenous drug use and was eventually admitted to an inpatient drug rehabilitation unit. He commenced treatment with buprenorphine to support his gradual withdrawal from opioid use (Figure 14.1).

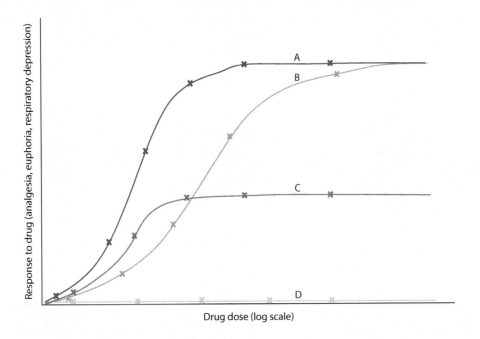

Figure 14.1 Dose-response curves.

Questions

1. The patient was treated with naloxone, and subsequently with buprenorphine. What is the mechanism of action of these two drugs?
2. This patient has been exposed to a number of drugs in the history relayed above, including heroin, fentanyl, buprenorphine and naloxone. Can you suggest which of these drugs are depicted in the dose-response curves A, B, C and D?

ANSWERS

1. Naloxone is a non-selective competitive μ-opioid receptor antagonist that can be administered by intravenous, intramuscular or nasal routes to treat opioid overdoses. Naloxone competitively binds to the μ-opioid receptor, thus preventing both endogenous and exogenous opioids from binding and exerting their effects. Naloxone is rapidly distributed and metabolised and thus has a rapid duration of effect. Patients with significant opioid toxicity may require multiple doses of naloxone, or even a continuous intravenous infusion to prevent respiratory depression.

   Buprenorphine is a partial agonist at the μ-opioid receptor that is prescribed to reduce dependence on opioids, such as heroin. The drug has a strong affinity for the μ-opioid receptor, competitively preventing other opioids from binding. Due to its partial agonist activity, buprenorphine does not induce significant pleasurable effects such as euphoria, in contrast with other opioids.

2. The dose-response curves show the potency and efficacy of the four drugs discussed: heroin, fentanyl, buprenorphine and naloxone. Drugs A and B are similarly efficacious, both achieving a similar level of response to the drugs. Drug A is more potent than Drug B however, meaning that smaller doses of Drug A are required to achieve maximal response compared with Drug B. In this scenario, Drug A is fentanyl, which is an extremely potent opioid that is commonly mixed with heroin, and small quantities of this drug can cause fatal overdoses. Drug B is heroin.

   Drug C is the partial μ-opioid receptor agonist, Buprenorphine, which is considerably less efficacious compared with fentanyl and heroin. Drug D is naloxone, the μ-opioid receptor antagonist that competes with other opioids and thus reduces their analgesic and depressive effects.

 Key Points

1. Naloxone is a non-selective competitive μ-opioid receptor antagonist that can be administered by intravenous, intramuscular or nasal routes to treat opioid overdoses.
2. Dose-response curves plot the biological response for a particular drug against the doses required to achieve that response. This allows us to assess and compare the efficacy and potency of drugs.

CASE 15: G-PROTEIN-COUPLED RECEPTORS

History

An 80-year-old woman presented to the emergency department with slurred speech and left arm weakness. Her symptoms had developed suddenly 12 h earlier and had gradually increased over the past 3 h. Her past medical history included hypertension, hypercholes-terolaemia and type 2 diabetes mellitus. Her regular medications were lercanidipine 10 mg OD, ramipril 5 mg OD, atorvastatin 40 mg ON and metformin 500 mg BD. She was a retired author, lived alone and was independent for all activities of daily living.

Examination

The patient was awake and alert. Her heart rate was 80 bpm and her blood pressure was 162/94 mmHg. On auscultation of her heart there was an ejection systolic murmur radiating to the carotids. Her chest was clear. Neurological examination identified no cranial nerve deficit and the patient agreed that her speech was no longer slurred. There was global weakness in the left upper limb with power of 4/5 throughout. There was subtle hypotonia of the left upper limb but reflexes were preserved. Sensation and co-ordination of the left upper limb were intact. Examination of the right upper limb and the lower limbs was unremarkable.

Results

A CT head scan showed ischaemia of the right middle cerebral artery territory.

Questions

1. Following the diagnosis of a right middle cerebral artery stroke, the patient was advised to commence anti-platelet therapy. Which anti-platelet agents are typically prescribed for the secondary prevention of stroke?
2. Clopidogrel exerts its anti-platelet actions by irreversibly binding to the $P2Y_{12}$ receptor, which is a 'G-protein-coupled receptor'. Describe the structure of a G-protein-coupled receptor.

ANSWERS

1. A variety of anti-platelet agents are used across the world in the secondary prevention of strokes and transient ischaemic attacks (TIA). In some centres, dipyridamole is prescribed alongside the COX-inhibitor, aspirin, whilst in other centres clopidogrel is prescribed as monotherapy.

   In the UK, The National Institute for Health and Care Excellence (NICE) recommends that clopidogrel be prescribed as the preferred treatment option for stroke, and that aspirin and dipyridamole dual therapy be prescribed for TIA prevention (clopidogrel is not currently licensed for this indication). The Royal College of Physicians recommends that clopidogrel monotherapy be prescribed as the treatment of choice for secondary prevention of both transient ischaemic attacks and strokes.

   Recent evidence suggests that patients who have sustained a minor ischemic stroke or high-risk TIA may benefit from dual anti-platelet therapy (aspirin and clopidogrel) for a short duration (up to 3 weeks) and future guidance may be changed to reflect this. Dual anti-platelet therapy is generally avoided in patients who have had a major stroke, due to the high risk of intracranial bleeding.

2. G-protein-coupled receptors are polypeptide receptors embedded within cell membranes, with an extracellular N-terminus, an intracellular C-terminus, and alpha helices that span the cell membrane seven times (see Figure 15.1), with an associated G-protein attached. The G-protein is heterotrimeric, consisting of alpha, beta and gamma subunits and is bound to GDP in its resting, inactive state.

   A vast variety of endogenous and synthetic ligands bind to the N-terminus of the G-protein-coupled receptor inducing a conformational change within the receptor. This activates the G-protein, causing GDP to be exchanged for GTP. The alpha subunit dissociates and activates other molecules, such as enzymes, within the cell. The beta-gamma dimer also interacts with other receptors within the cell, including ion channels. Once the GTP is hydrolysed to GDP, the G-protein inactivates and reforms alongside the G-protein-coupled receptor.

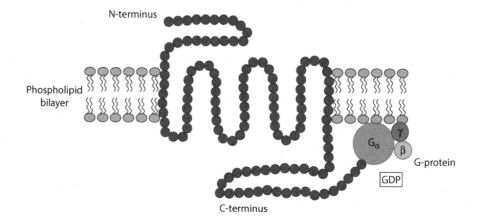

Figure 15.1 A G-protein-coupled receptor.

G-protein-coupled receptors are prolific in eukaryotes, with approximately 1000 different types identified thus far in humans. G-protein-coupled receptors are common pharmaceutical targets and over a third of medicines currently approved by the US Food and Drug Administration exert their mechanisms of action via G-protein-coupled receptors.

🔑	Key Points
	1. G-protein-coupled receptors are polypeptide receptors embedded within cell membranes, to which a wide variety of endogenous and synthetic ligands bind.
	2. Over a third of currently licensed drugs target G-protein-coupled receptors.

SECTION 2
THERAPEUTICS

History

A 24-year-old man presented to hospital via ambulance after being found unconscious at a party. He was found to have a small bottle of clear, colourless liquid in his pocket. His friend reported that this was 'GHB'. It was unclear whether the patient had co-ingested other recreational drugs or alcohol.

Examination

The patient was drowsy but maintaining his own airway. His eyes opened to painful stimuli, he made localised movements in response to painful stimuli and he replied to speech with inappropriate words (Glasgow Coma Scale = 10 points). Systemic examination was otherwise unremarkable.

Results

Routine blood tests were unremarkable. An ECG showed normal sinus rhythm.

Questions

1. What is 'GHB'?
2. How should this patient be managed?

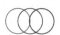

ANSWERS

1. Gamma-hydroxybutyric acid (GHB) and its prodrug, gamma-butyrolactone (GBL), are psychoactive drugs with sedative effects. They are usually sold as small bottles or vials of colourless liquids that are taken orally. Frequent recreational use of GHB/GBL may result in physical dependence. Regular users of GHB/GBL will typically measure out precise volumes of the liquid using syringes to prevent overdosing.

2. The patient should be managed in a clinical area with staff who can provide airway support. As with any patient with reduced consciousness, routine assessments including a full systemic examination, basic blood tests (a blood glucose level, full blood count, renal profile, and C-reactive protein level) should be carried out and if there is any suspicion of opioid use, naloxone (an opioid receptor antagonist) should be given intravenously. Patients with GHB/GBL dependence may subsequently develop symptoms of withdrawal, including agitation, confusion and hallucinations. Such patients may require high doses of benzodiazepines to manage their agitation, or even sedation with intubation and ventilation, and thus should be discussed with local or national clinical toxicologists who will guide further management.

CASE 17: ECSTASY

History

A 17-year-old woman was brought to the emergency department after collapsing at a night-club. Her friend reported that she had taken an ecstasy tablet 2 h earlier. The patient's friend stated that they had both consumed alcohol but denied the use of other recreational drugs. The patient had a witnessed tonic clonic seizure shortly after the ambulance service arrived.

Examination

The patient's temperature was elevated at 38.2°C. She was drowsy but roused to pain. She was tachycardic with a heart rate of 170 beats per minute. Her blood pressure was 122/70 mmHg. Her respiratory rate was elevated at 32 breaths per minute but her chest was clear to auscultation.

Results

Bloods: WCC 14.4 (neutrophil count 12.0, lymphocyte count 2.1), Hb 120, Plt 460, Na 131, K 3.7, Creat 70, CK 7400

Questions

1. What clinical sequelae can result from ecstasy toxicity?
2. How should this patient be managed?

ANSWERS

1. Ecstasy or 3,4-methylenedioxymethamphetamine (MDMA) is an amphetamine derivative that continues to be one of the most commonly used recreational drugs worldwide. The drug enhances the pre-synaptic release of serotonin, dopamine and noradrenaline.

   The anticipated effects of ecstasy include a sense of euphoria and relaxation, whilst adverse effects can range from dehydration to seizures. Elevated serotonin levels can result in severe tachycardia, hyperpyrexia, rhabdomyolysis, the development of a metabolic acidosis, renal failure and disseminated intravascular coagulation. Patients with prominent serotonergic symptoms and signs are at risk of significant morbidity and mortality.

2. Patients with mild toxicity may only require basic supportive measures such as intravenous fluid rehydration. Benzodiazepines may be required to manage agitation or myoclonus. Patients with severe serotonin syndrome will need further management in a critical care environment to provide cardiovascular and/or respiratory support.

   Active cooling mechanisms, such as applying ice packs externally or cooled intravenous fluids, should be used to treat hyperpyrexia. Cyproheptadine, a 5-HT2 receptor antagonist, should be administered although this is only available in a tablet form and, thus a nasogastric tube may need to be sited if the patient is unable to swallow medication. Renal replacement therapy may also be required if the patient develops significant rhabdomyolysis alongside an acute kidney injury.

History

A 78-year-old man was brought to hospital by his family after developing symptoms of nausea and vomiting. He had been vomiting intermittently for the preceding 24 h and was unable to tolerate oral fluids. He also reported several episodes of diarrhoea, passing watery green-brown stools on each occasion.

The patient had been feeling well until the onset of the vomiting and had experienced no recent illnesses. Of note, he had not received any courses of antibiotics recently. His granddaughter had experienced similar symptoms of diarrhoea and vomiting 3–4 days earlier.

Examination

The patient appeared generally well although his mucus membranes were dry. His blood pressure was 100/70 mHg and his heart rate was 102 beats per minute. His abdomen was soft and non-tender throughout with normal bowel sounds.

Results

Bloods: WCC 14.2 (neutrophils 11.3, lymphocytes 2.5), Hb 123, MCV 85, Plt 350, Na 134, K 3.6, Creat 120 (baseline 80), CRP 46, Blood glucose 5.4

Questions

1. What is the most probable diagnosis?
2. Which medications should be prescribed to treat the patient's nausea and vomiting?

ANSWERS

1. The differential diagnosis for nausea and vomiting is broad. There is no history of progressive swallowing difficulties, odynophagia or regurgitation, thus making a structural lesion within the oesophagus unlikely. There is additionally no abdominal pain on examination and the bowel sounds are normal and thus bowel obstruction is also unlikely. Neurological causes of vomiting, such as a space-occupying lesion should be considered, although such cases typically present with worsening symptoms after sleeping and may have associated changes in mental status.

   The patient's blood results show elevated inflammatory markers (raised white cell count and CRP) and an acute kidney injury (creatinine level greater than 150% of baseline) and this is suggestive of a diagnosis of infection and pre-renal failure secondary to vomiting and diarrhoea. Gastroenteritis is the most probable diagnosis, particularly in view of the patient's granddaughter experiencing similar symptoms recently. The patient has not received antibiotics recently and *Clostridium difficile* infection is therefore unlikely. Other infections, such as lower respiratory tract or urinary tract infections should also be considered, although these are less likely.

2. The patient should be prescribed an anti-emetic, either orally (if tolerated), or intravenously. The intramuscular or subcutaneous routes are also an option for some anti-emetics. The most commonly prescribed agents include:

   a. Ondansetron, a serotonin 5-HT3 antagonist, which acts on the chemoreceptor trigger zone in the medulla oblungata. This drug is particularly efficacious in chemotherapy-induced vomiting.

   b. Cyclizine and cinnarizine, histamine H1 receptor antagonists, which are thought to also act on the chemoreceptor trigger zone and are particularly useful in the management of vomiting induced by vertigo or motion sickness.

   c. Metoclopramide, a dopamine D_2 antagonist, that additionally acts on the chemoreceptor trigger zone. This drug also displays 5-HT4 receptor agonist activity. Metoclopramide is prokinetic and promotes gastric emptying, which may also contribute to its anti-emetic effect.

CASE 19: MANAGING PAIN

History

A 52-year-old man was admitted to hospital with a pleural effusion of unknown aetiology. A chest drain was sited during his hospital stay and he now complains of moderate pain around the chest wall, following the drain insertion. His past medical history included peptic ulcer disease with two previous upper gastrointestinal bleeds. His regular medications include omeprazole 40 mg OD.

Examination

On examination, the patient appears comfortable at rest and there is no tachypnoea or obvious dyspnoea. There is reduced air entry at the right lung base, which is also dull to percussion. The water level in the drain rises and falls with inspiration and expiration, respectively.

Results

A chest X-ray, performed shortly after the above examination shows a small residual pleural effusion with no pneumothorax.

Questions

1. The patient is requesting analgesia but declines paracetamol as he thinks this is 'not strong enough'. What should you prescribe for him?
2. The patient requests naproxen, as he has heard from another patient on the ward that this is a good analgesic agent. Is this an appropriate choice of analgesia?

ANSWERS

1. The first-line agents in the traditional analgesic ladder are simple analgesics, such as paracetamol. This can be prescribed regularly in patients with moderate to severe pain. Weak opioids, such as codeine phosphate and dihydrocodeine, are typically prescribed as second-line analgesics for moderate to severe pain. Stronger opioids, such as morphine, are prescribed for severe pain. In cases of neuropathic pain, agents such as gabapentin (a gabapentinoid), pregabalin (a gabapentinoid) and amitriptyline (a tricyclic antidepressant) may be beneficial.

   There is good evidence in the medical literature to support the use of paracetamol in moderate-to-severe pain, as regular paracetamol (four times daily) can provide 'background' analgesic effects. Multiple studies show that the combination of paracetamol and opioids produces an additive analgesic effect, and this patient should initially be given paracetamol regularly, along with a weak opioid as required.

2. The patient has a past medical history that includes previous upper gastrointestinal bleeding. Non-steroidal anti-inflammatory drugs (NSAIDs) are effective analgesic and anti-pyretic agents but can have significant adverse effects. NSAIDs inhibit the cyclo-oxygenase (COX) enzyme, leading to a reduction in prostaglandin synthesis. Prostaglandins have many biological functions, including inhibition of acid secretion from gastric parietal cells and increased gastrointestinal mucus secretion. NSAIDs, such as diclofenac, can therefore increase the risk of gastrointestinal bleeding and should be avoided in patients with a history of gastritis or peptic ulcer disease, where possible.

History

An 83-year-old woman was admitted to hospital with shortness of breath and fever. She was diagnosed with a community-acquired pneumonia and was treated with intravenous antibiotics. Despite being lucid throughout the day, she became agitated and confused overnight. The following morning, the patient's mental state and cognition had returned to baseline. The patient had no history of dementia or cognitive impairment. Her past history was significant for hypertension and a previous hip replacement. Her regular medications were ramipril 2.5 mg OD and paracetamol 1 g QDS PRN. She lived alone and was independent with all activities of daily living. She did not drink alcohol and had never smoked.

Examination

The patient was examined whilst she was confused. She was alert and agitated. She was not orientated to time or place but was orientated to person. Cardiovascular, respiratory, abdominal and neurological examinations were unremarkable.

Results

Bloods: WCC 11.6 (neutrophils 8.1), Hb 102, MCV 83, Plt 344, Na 140, K 4.1, Creat 65, CRP 72

Questions

1. Which investigations should be considered to identify a cause for the patient's transient confusion?
2. If the patient becomes confused and agitated again, which medications could be prescribed to manage this?

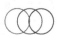

ANSWERS

1. The patient has fluctuating confusion consistent with delirium. Infection is a common precipitant for delirium and, in this case, the patient has an underlying pneumonia. Where infection is suspected as a cause for delirium, blood tests should be sent to identify possible raised inflammatory markers. Blood cultures should be considered, particularly if the patient is febrile and investigations such as a sputum culture, urine dip, stool sample for microscopy and culture if there is diarrhoea, and a chest X-ray should be considered.

    Electrolyte abnormalities, particularly hyper- and hyponatraemia, hyper- and hypoglycaemia, and hypercalcaemia, are common causes of confusion, and these should therefore be checked. Hyper- and hypothyroidism can also lead to cognitive impairment, and a thyroid stimulating hormone level should therefore be measured.

    If there is a history of preceding trauma such as a fall that resulted in a head injury, or if the patient is taking anticoagulant medications, then a CT scan of the head should be considered to exclude an intracranial bleed.

2. It is important to emphasise that non-pharmacological methods of managing delirium, such as nursing patients in a quiet, dimly lit environment with continuity of care from staff, is always preferable. Where patients are at risk of harming themselves or others and de-escalation techniques have failed, pharmacological management should be commenced.

    Firstly, drugs that may exacerbate delirium, including psychoactive medications, should need to be discontinued where possible. Secondly, drugs to treat agitation may need to be prescribed. Administering a low dose, observing the effect and then prescribing a further dose if needed is safer than starting with a higher dose.

    Antipsychotic medications, such as haloperidol and olanzapine, are usually the first-line therapy, although they can prolong the QT interval, and a baseline ECG should therefore be reviewed prior to prescribing these drugs. Adverse effects of antipsychotic medications also include extra-pyramidal symptoms and they should thus be avoided in patients with Parkinson's disease or Lewy body dementia. Benzodiazepines are generally accepted as the second-line agent of choice to manage delirium and are particularly recommended for the treatment of delirium tremens.

History

A 24-year-old woman visits hospital reporting that she took a paracetamol overdose 4 h earlier in an attempt to end her life. The patient describes taking 32 × 500 mg paracetamol tablets. She took the tablets all at once, over a 5-min period. She was certain of the time of the overdose, as she checked her phone and sent a text message as she was taking the tablets. She did not take any other medications or any recreational drugs with the paracetamol and did not drink any alcohol at the time. Her past medical history included a diagnosis of depression, for which she was taking sertraline 50 mg OD. She took no other regular medications and had no known drug allergies. She was a postgraduate university student, drank approximately 14 units of alcohol per week and did not use recreational drugs.

Examination

Systems examination was unremarkable.

Results

Bloods: Na 138, K 3.8, Creat 50, Bili 4, ALT 11, ALP 40, INR 1.0, Paracetamol concentration 150 mg/L

Questions

1. Describe how paracetamol is metabolised.
2. Based on the above results, how should this patient be managed?

ANSWERS

1. Paracetamol is metabolised in the liver. It is predominantly conjugated into glucuronide and sulphate conjugates. A small proportion of the paracetamol is metabolised by cytochrome P_{450} enzymes (mainly CYP2E1 and CYP3A4) into the toxic metabolite, N-acetyl-p-benzoquinoneimine (NAPQI). When there are adequate stores of the anti-oxidant, glutathione, NAPQI is conjugated to form non-toxic metabolites (Figure 21.1).

   In the case of paracetamol overdose, the initial conjugation pathway is exceeded and greater production of NAPQI occurs. Glutathione stores become depleted and NAPQI concentrations accumulate resulting in hepatocyte damage and potentially the development of fulminant liver failure (Figure 21.2).

   Acetylcysteine is converted to cysteine in the gastrointestinal system, and cysteine is a constituent of glutathione. Acetylcysteine thus replenishes glutathione stores, allowing NAPQI to be metabolised, preventing further liver damage.

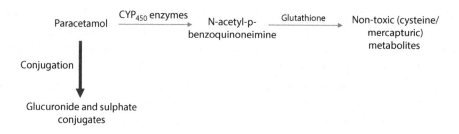

Figure 21.1 Normal paracetamol metabolism.

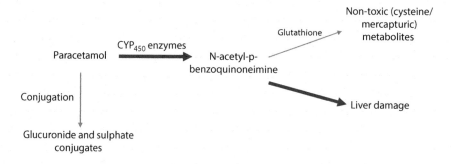

Figure 21.2 Paracetamol metabolism in overdose.

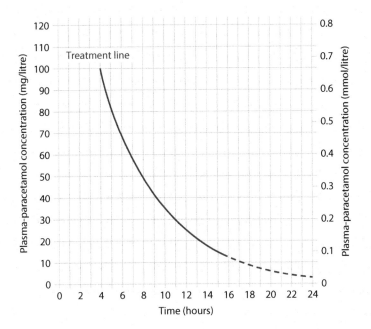

Figure 21.3 Revised paracetamol overdose treatment nomogram. (Image taken from Royal College of Emergency Medicine website – https://www.rcem.ac.uk/.)

2. According to the Royal College of Emergency Medicine guidelines, and in keeping with similar guidance from across the world, significant paracetamol overdoses should be treated with a course of acetylcysteine. Patients who present within an hour of the overdose should also be given activated charcoal – this is a form of carbon that has a large surface area and thus adsorbs many toxins.

   In the United Kingdom, we use the nomogram shown in Figure 21.3 to guide decisions regarding the treatment of paracetamol overdoses. The data is only accurate from 4 to 16 h, and a serum paracetamol concentration is therefore uninterpretable until 4 h post-overdose. Acetylcysteine may be commenced prior to the result becoming available if the patient has taken a large overdose, for example, >150 mg/kg.

   If the patient's serum paracetamol concentration falls within 10% of the nomogram treatment line, or the patient is uncertain of the timing of their overdose, the safest option is to treat them with a course of acetylcysteine.

   Following treatment with acetylcysteine, the patient should have repeat blood tests performed to check if their renal and liver function (LFTs and INR) is satisfactory. If there is significant renal or liver impairment, a further infusion of acetylcysteine may need to be commenced. Patients with severe hepatic dysfunction should be referred to the local liver unit for consideration of a liver transplant.

History
An 81-year-old woman was brought to hospital by her family after she complained of drowsiness and shortness of breath. Her past medical history included breast cancer with metastases to the brain, liver and bones. She had undergone a mastectomy with lymph node clearance, received 3 cycles of chemotherapy and had undergone several sessions of targeted radiotherapy. At her last oncology appointment, she was advised that further active treatment would not be appropriate and she was referred to the community palliative care team. Her regular medications were: dexamethasone 8mg PO BD, paracetamol 1 g PO QDS, dihydrocodeine 30 mg PO QDS and morphine sulphate immediate release oral solution 5–10 mg up to 4 hourly. She lived with her husband, did not drink alcohol and was an ex-smoker with a 40-pack-year history.

Examination
The patient was drowsy but alert to pain. She appeared cachectic. Her heart rate was 100 bpm and her blood pressure was 96/60 mmHg. There were coarse crackles heard bilaterally throughout her chest and there was bronchial breathing over the left mid-zone and right upper-zone. Her abdomen was soft and non-tender. Her pupils were 4 mm bilaterally and there were no focal neurological signs.

Results
Bloods: WCC 15.4, Hb 92, Plt 572, Na 132, K 6.1, Creat 320, CRP 320

CT brain: progression of known metastatic disease

Questions
1. The palliative care team feel that the patient is approaching the final days of her life and advise that anticipatory medicines be prescribed. What are 'anticipatory medicines'?
2. If the patient requires multiple doses of anticipatory medicines, how can their symptoms be more effectively managed?

ANSWERS

1. The patient is in pain and is becoming increasingly drowsy. To ensure that the end of her life is comfortable and dignified, several 'as needed' medications should be prescribed so that there is no unnecessary delay to treating any symptoms that should arise.

   The medications should be prescribed to be administered subcutaneously. The subcutaneous route is often more appropriate than the oral route towards the end of a patient's life, as dying patients are often drowsy and may not be able to swallow safely. Gastrointestinal absorption and bowel motility also deteriorates as patients develop multi-organ failure. The intravenous route requires a cannula *in situ* for delivery – patients may be oedematous and it can be challenging to establish intravenous access in a timely fashion. Additionally, multiple attempts at venous cannulation is painful and may distress the patient.

   Even if the patient is comfortable at the time of assessment, you should prescribe medications to control four potential symptoms and signs:
   a. Pain – morphine is usually the drug of choice. Alfentanil may be used in renal disease
   b. Nausea and vomiting – haloperidol or levomepromazine are appropriate options
   c. Agitation and breathlessness – haloperidol usually the drug of choice
   d. Increased respiratory secretions – glycopyrronium or hyoscine are appropriate options

2. If a patient requires more than three doses of a single anticipatory medicine or if two or more medicines are required within 24 h, then a syringe pump should be considered. This prevents multiple subcutaneous injections from being administered and delivers a constant background dose of anticipatory medicines that can be titrated according to response.

   Once a syringe pump is established, further use of breakthrough anticipatory medicines will be assessed over the next 12-h period and the pump will then be adjusted as needed. The palliative care team are often able to provide support with setting up and adjusting a syringe pump.

History

A 74-year-old woman was reviewed routinely by her general practitioner. She had been well recently but her daughter, who is the patient's main carer, had been struggling to administer her daily medications. The patient had advanced Alzheimer's dementia and was often reluctant to take oral medications. Her daughter wondered if all of the medications were necessary. The patient's past medical history included the aforementioned Alzheimer's dementia, frequent falls (one of which resulted in a previous fracture of the left neck of femur), Parkinson's disease, hypercholesterolaemia, hypertension and type-2 diabetes mellitus. Her regular medications were: co-careldopa 50/200 mg PO TDS, aspirin 75 mg PO OD, atorvastatin 20 mg PO ON, omeprazole 20 mg PO OD, doxazosin 4 mg PO BD, ramipril 5 mg PO OD and metformin 1 g PO BD.

Examination

The patient appeared frail and tremulous. She was mobilising unsteadily around the room. Her heart rate was 70 bpm and her blood pressure was 120/80 mmHg. Her chest was clear and her abdomen was soft and non-tender.

Questions

1. What is de-prescribing?
2. Which of the patient's medications could potentially be 'de-prescribed'?

ANSWERS

1. De-prescribing is the process of reviewing regular medications in older adults and assessing what drugs could be withdrawn with the aim of improving patient outcomes. Data shows that older adults are being prescribed increasing quantities of medications as they develop further co-morbidities. Many medications will cause adverse effects, for which further medications are added in.

   Data suggests that patients in the final year of their life are prescribed an average of 10–12 medications daily. Polypharmacy comes with significant burdens in terms of drug interactions, adverse effects, financial costs, as well as the inconvenience for the patient who has to take multiple tablets. De-prescribing attempts to balance the benefits of taking each prescribed medication with the potential negative aspects of this, and to then decide whether the patient is ultimately likely to derive significant benefit from this medication.

2. Based on the patient's past medical history, atorvastatin appears to be used for primary cardiovascular prevention in this case. It would be reasonable to stop this medication at this point in the patient's life.

   It is unclear why the patient is taking aspirin – this should be reviewed. If the patient is not taking this for secondary prevention of cardiovascular disease, it would be reasonable to consider stopping this. It may then be that the patient will not need to take her omeprazole if this was prescribed for aspirin-induced gastritis.

   Metformin may be important to keep on the prescription – the patient may be at risk of developing significant hyperglycaemia if this is stopped. The patient's recent HbA1c levels should be reviewed to assess her recent glycaemic control. Patients with Alzheimer's dementia often eat progressively smaller amounts of food as their disease progresses and thus their carbohydrate intake declines. The patient may require a reduced dose of metformin to manage her glycaemic control or may even be able to stop this medication. In some cases, where patients are frail with multiple comorbidities, physicians and patients agree to target a less rigid glucose range, for example, 4–12 mmol/L.

   According to the aforementioned history, the patient has had multiple falls recently, one of which has resulted in a fracture. Her blood pressure control should be reviewed and one or both of her antihypertensive agents should be ceased. If there is an element of postural hypotension making falls more likely, then it may be considered safer, on balance, to stop the antihypertensives if this reduces the patient's risk of falling.

   Co-careldopa (carbidopa and levodopa) is likely to prevent significant Parkinson's disease symptoms and this should therefore be continued. Stiffness and bradycardia will increase her risk of falling and will likely cause distress and agitation.

   The physician caring for the patient should continue to review the patient after introducing any changes to her prescription – for example, she may develop symptoms after ceasing certain medications, or her blood pressure and glycaemic control could worsen. As with all patients, it is important to review her regular medications whenever the opportunity arises.

History

A 29-year-old woman attended her general practitioner and explained that she wanted to plan a pregnancy. Her past medical history is significant for epilepsy. Her epilepsy had been poorly controlled during her teenage years but had been relatively stable for 10 years on sodium valproate. She experienced a tonic-clonic seizure approximately 2–3 times per year. Her regular medications were sodium valproate 600 mg BD and the combined oral contraceptive pill. She worked as an illustrator and lived with her partner. She did not drink alcohol and had never smoked.

Questions

1. How will you counsel the patient with regards to planning a pregnancy in view of her medical history?
2. Which therapeutic options are available to the patient to manage her epilepsy during pregnancy?

ANSWERS

1. Epilepsy control often declines during pregnancy. Women experience significant fluctuations in oral intake, gastrointestinal absorption, hormone levels, fluid status, cardiovascular output and renal function, all of which lead to altered circulating antiepileptic drug levels. Significant psychosocial stressors also arise and patients may experience poor sleep, further impairing epileptic control. As a result, patients are more likely to have seizures during pregnancy and should be regularly reviewed with regards to their epilepsy throughout the pregnancy.

   Antiepileptic drugs are associated with significant adverse effects and several of them appear to affect foetal development. Sodium valproate, carbamazepine and phenytoin are associated with an increased risk of developing congenital abnormalities. Sodium valproate, in particular, is associated with major congenital abnormalities, including a 20-fold increase in neural tube defects, as well as cardiovascular abnormalities and cleft palate. Sodium valproate exposure in pregnancy is also associated with reduced intelligence quotient and verbal quotient scores in childhood, as well as an increased risk of autism.

2. Recent guidance from the UK Medicines and Healthcare Products Regulatory Agency (MHRA) advises that women and girls of childbearing potential should not be prescribed sodium valproate unless they are using a form of highly effective contraception (an intrauterine device [IUD], an intrauterine system [IUS], the hormonal injection, the progestogen-only implant and sterilisation).

   Sodium valproate is a very effective anti-epileptic drug and it may be the case that other treatments will be less effective in achieving seizure control and that, on balance, the risk of having frequent tonic-clonic seizures outweighs the risk to foetal development. Nevertheless, there are a variety of antiepileptic drugs that may be suitable for the patient. Whilst data are limited, it appears that carbamazepine and lamotrigine monotherapy at the lower doses have the least risk of congenital abnormalities. Meaningful data in relation to safety in pregnancy is lacking for newer agents, such as levitaracetam.

   Ultimately, the patient should avoid pregnancy whilst taking sodium valproate, if possible. The patient should be referred to a specialist epilepsy clinic where the neurology team can provide further information regarding her treatment options. The patient should be advised to continue both the sodium valproate and the contraception prior to this review.

History

A 42-year-old woman presented to the emergency department after becoming light-headed and short of breath when rushing to work. Her symptoms had fully resolved by the time she was reviewed by a physician. She described feeling increasingly fatigued over recent weeks. She had no known past medical history and took no regular medications. The patient worked as a caterer, did not drink alcohol and had never smoked.

Examination

The patient appeared clinically well, although there was visible conjunctival pallor. Her heart sounds were dual with no murmurs, her heart rate was 90 bpm and her blood pressure was 126/74 mmHg. Her chest was clear, her respiratory rate was 14 breaths per minute and her peripheral oxygen saturations were 98% on room air. Her abdomen was soft and non-tender with no palpable masses. There was no peripheral oedema. Neurological examination was unremarkable.

Results

Bloods: WCC 5.2, Hb 88, MCV 114, Plt 280, Na 139, K 4.0, Creat 47, CRP < 1

Questions

1. What are the potential causes of the abnormal findings reported above?
2. What pharmacological treatment options may be available for the patient?

ANSWERS

1. The patient has presented with symptoms of fatigue and light-headedness and her blood results show a macrocytic anaemia. The most common causes of macrocytic anaemia are:
   a. Folate deficiency
   b. B_{12} deficiency
   c. Functional B_{12} deficiency

   Folate deficiency typically develops due to dietary deficiencies or malabsorption, including coeliac disease. Folate deficiency may also occur in patients who have an increase in folate requirements, such as occurs in pregnancy. Folate deficiencies have also been linked to the use of tanning beds, although the potential mechanism underlying this is unclear.

   B_{12} deficiency also develops due to nutritional deficiencies, such as a poor diet or alcoholism, and due to malabsorption. Pernicious anaemia is the most common cause of B_{12} deficiency in the United Kingdom. For patients with low-normal B12 levels, methylmalonic acid is a more sensitive marker of B12 deficiency.

   Functional B_{12} deficiency can occur following nitrous oxide exposure as the cobalt within B_{12} becomes irreversibly oxidised, rendering vitamin B_{12} inactive. In these cases, homocysteine levels accumulate (elevated homocysteine levels can be used as a marker for functional B_{12} deficiency). Patients with chronic nitrous oxide exposure are at risk of developing subacute combined degeneration of the cord. This can occur due to recreational use of nitrous oxide or when this is prescribed in hospital as a form of analgesia, for example, in patients in labour or with sickle cell crises.

   The patient's blood should be sent to measure vitamin B_{12}, methylmalonic acid and folic acid concentrations to guide further investigations and management.

2. If the patient has a vitamin B_{12} or folic acid deficiency, these can be replaced through pharmacological therapies. Folic acid can be prescribed as a once-daily 5 mg oral dose. Vitamin B_{12} is typically replaced via a series of intramuscular hydroxocobalamin injections, initially prescribed as 1 mg 3 times a week for 2 weeks, then 1 mg every 2–3 months. Cyanocobalamin is an oral formulation of vitamin B_{12} that can be prescribed at doses of 50–150 µg daily.

   It was previously thought that patients who were deficient in both B_{12} and folic acid needed to have the B_{12} replaced first or they would be at increased risk of developing subacute combined degeneration of the cord. More recent data does not suggest that this is the case and patients typically receive folic acid and B_{12} replacement together without consequence.

SECTION 3
PRESCRIBING CASES

History

A 23-year-old woman presented to hospital with a 24-h history of headache and fever. The headache was global, had come on gradually and was now severe. The patient had been feeling unwell since the past day and described episodes of feeling cold and shivery. She complained that light caused discomfort to her eyes and she was thus holding a scarf over her face. The patient had vomited several times.

She had no past medical history, did not take any regular medications and had no known drug allergies.

Examination

The patient was febrile at 38.6°C. Her heart rate was 110 bpm and her blood pressure was 106/60 mmHg. She was photophobic and Kernig's sign was positive.

Question

Using the once-only side of the drug chart below, please prescribe the first medication that should be administered to the patient.

ONCE ONLY MEDICATIONS									
Date	Medication	Dose	Route	Time of dose	Signature	Prescriber	Given by	Time given	Pharmacy

ANSWER

ONCE ONLY MEDICATIONS									
Date	Medication	Dose	Route	Time of dose	Signature	Prescriber	Given by	Time given	Pharmacy
01/01/20	CEFTRIAXONE	2 g	IV	12:00	*A Doctor*	A DOCTOR			

The patient has symptoms and signs consistent with meningitis – this could be viral, bacterial, fungal or autoimmune in origin. If bacterial meningitis or meningococcal septicaemia are suspected, antibiotic therapy should be started as soon as possible as morbidity and mortality rates from these conditions are very high.

Ceftriaxone is typically the first-line treatment to treat bacterial meningitis, although other broad-spectrum cephalosporins with good bactericidal activity in the cerebrospinal fluid may also be appropriate. The first dose of this is usually 1–2 g given intravenously.

Patients with a past history of anaphylaxis to penicillins will need to be treated with an alternative antibiotic – this should be discussed with a microbiology specialist to ensure adequate antibiotic coverage is provided.

History

A 70-year-old woman was admitted to hospital following a fall. She was unable to provide history regarding the fall and the doctor assessing her reported that she was confused. Her past medical history included gastro-oesophageal reflux disease, depression, hypertension, hypercholesterolaemia and heart failure. Her medications are listed below. She lived alone, was reportedly independent with all activities of daily living, and usually volunteered at a local charity shop. She did not drink alcohol, did not use recreational drugs and had never smoked.

Examination

Systems examination was unremarkable and the patient looked clinically well and appeared euvolaemic. She was not orientated to time or place but was aware of her name, age and date of birth.

Results

Bloods: WCC 6.2, Hb 120, Plt 340, Na 120, K 3.8, Creat 59, CRP < 1

Question

Which four medications are most likely to be responsible for the abnormality in her blood results, as shown above?

Amlodipine	5 mg	PO	OD	☐
Atorvastatin	40 mg	PO	ON	☐
Carbamazepine	200 mg	PO	BD	☐
Furosemide	40 mg	PO	BD	☐
Omeprazole	40 mg	PO	OD	☐
Paracetamol	1 g	PO	QDS	☐
Sertraline	50 mg	PO	OD	☐
Temazepam	10 mg	PO	ON	☐

ANSWER

Amlodipine	5 mg	PO	OD	☐
Atorvastatin	40 mg	PO	ON	☐
Carbamazepine	200 mg	PO	BD	X
Furosemide	40 mg	PO	BD	X
Omeprazole	40 mg	PO	OD	X
Paracetamol	1 g	PO	QDS	☐
Sertraline	50 mg	PO	OD	X
Temazepam	10 mg	PO	ON	☐

The patient's blood results show hyponatraemia. Numerous classes of drugs can cause hyponatraemia, and both thiazide and loop diuretics (furosemide) are agents that are commonly responsible. Thiazide diuretics act by inhibiting reabsorption of sodium from the distal convoluted tubule whilst loop diuretics inhibit sodium transport in the renal medulla, thus increasing sodium excretion.

Selective serotonin-reuptake inhibitors (sertraline) and some anti-epileptic drugs (carbamazepine) can cause hyponatraemia by inducing excessive production of the anti-diuretic hormone (ADH) resulting in the syndrome of inappropriate ADH release (SIADH). ADH promotes re-absorption of water back into the circulation, thus reducing the circulating osmolality. Drug-induced SIADH is a common cause of hyponatraemia.

The mechanism by which protein pump inhibitors (omeprazole) induce hyponatraemia is unclear but is thought to be related to an excessive loss of urinary sodium.

History

A 35-year-old man was being treated in hospital for a community-acquired pneumonia. He was receiving intravenous antibiotics and was likely to be in hospital for more than 24 h. The patient had no past medical history, took no regular medications and had no known drug allergies.

The patient drank approximately 1 L of vodka daily plus 2–4 cans of strong lager (approximately 50 units of alcohol per day). After 6 h in hospital, he became tremulous and sweaty and his nurse reported concerns that he is withdrawing from alcohol.

Results

Bloods: WCC 14.2, Hb 140, Plt 220, Na 138, K 4.2, Creat 70, CRP 80, Bili 14, ALT 35, ALP 52, INR 1.1

Question

Using the 'as needed' drug chart below, prescribe one medication to treat his symptoms of alcohol withdrawal. On the 'regular medications' drug chart, prescribe one medication to help prevent the patient from developing Wernicke's encephalopathy.

'As needed' medications

DRUG (print approved name)		Dose	Date					
			Time					
Signature	Date	Route	Dose					
Print name	Bleep	Pharmacy	Route					
Indication/additional information		Max dose freq	Name					

Regular medications

			Date					
DRUG (print approved name)		Dose	6					
			8					
Signature	Date	Route	12					
Print name	Bleep	Pharmacy	14					
			18					
Additional information			22					

ANSWER

'As needed' medications

DRUG (print approved name)		Dose	Date						
CHLORDIAZEPOXIDE		25–50 mg	Time						
Signature *A DOCTOR*	Date 01/01/2020	Route PO	Dose						
Print name A DOCTOR	Bleep 1234	Pharmacy	Route						
Indication/additional information As per CIWA-Ar score		Max dose freq 2 HOURLY	Name						

Regular medications

			Date						
DRUG (print approved name)		Dose	6						
PABRINEX		1 PAIR	(8)						
Signature *A DOCTOR*	Date 01/01/2020	Route 01/01/2020	12						
Print name A DOCTOR	Bleep 1234	Pharmacy	(14)						
Additional information			18						
			(22)						

This patient drinks at least 50 units of alcohol per day and is thus at significant risk of developing symptoms and signs of alcohol withdrawal. Patients who have their alcohol intake abruptly ceased or reduced can become tremulous, agitated and may ultimately develop seizures or delirium tremens.

Benzodiazepines should be prescribed to manage acute alcohol withdrawal. Chlordiazepoxide is typically the benzodiazepine of choice as it has a relatively low potential for abuse. This is prescribed orally. Patients with impaired liver function should be treated with either a reduced dose of chlordiazepoxide or lorazepam. Intravenous diazepam or lorazepam may be indicated if urgent control is required. This patient does not have significantly impaired liver function, as indicated by his normal liver function tests and INR result. The dose and frequency of benzodiazepines required is usually determined using an objective withdrawal scoring system, such as the 'Clinical Institute Withdrawal Assessment of Alcohol Scale, Revised (CIWA-Ar)', to identify signs of withdrawal, such as tremor.

A parenteral preparation of vitamins B and C, such as Pabrinex®, containing thiamine, riboflavin, pyridoxine, nicotinamide and ascorbic acid should be prescribed to prevent the development of Wernicke's encephalopathy in patients who are considered to be at risk of withdrawing from alcohol. Higher doses of this preparation should be provided for those who are thought to have developed Wernicke's encephalopathy.

History

A 68-year-old woman presented to hospital with a 3-day history of shortness of breath and a dry cough. Her past medical history included chronic obstructive pulmonary disease (COPD). Her only regular medications are a salbutamol inhaler and a corticosteroid inhaler. She had no known drug allergies.

Examination

On examination, the patient's respiratory rate was 26 and there was a widespread polyphonic wheeze heard throughout her chest. Her peripheral oxygen saturations (SpO_2) were 86% on room air.

Results

Bloods: WCC 7.8, Hb 121, Plt 250, CRP 4, Chest X-ray – hyperexpanded lung fields

An arterial blood gas shows: pH 7.37, pCO_2 6.5, pO_2 8.0, HCO_3 32, BE 0.2

Question

Based on the information above, please prescribe oxygen for this patient using the chart below.

CONTINUOUS OXYGEN PRESCRIPTION CHART

PATIENT DETAILS (affix sticker)						
Given name						
Family name						
Patient ID						
DOB						
Sex M☐ F☐						

Start date/time	Target oxygen saturations (circle)	Current device/flow rate	Prescriber name	Prescriber signature	Prescriber position/ bleep no.
	94–98%				
	88–92%				
	Palliative use				

In an emergency, all patients should receive high flow oxygen immediately if required

ANSWER

CONTINUOUS OXYGEN PRESCRIPTION CHART

PATIENT DETAILS (affix sticker)	
Given name	Anne
Family name	Patient
Patient ID	123456A
DOB	01/01/1952
Sex	M ☐ F ☒

Start date/time	Target oxygen saturations (circle)	Current device/flow rate	Prescriber name	Prescriber signature	Prescriber position/ bleep no.
01/01/2020 12:00	~~94–98%~~ (88–92%) Palliative use	Venturi 24% set at 2L per minute	A. DOCTOR	*A Doctor*	FY1 doctor 1234

In an emergency, all patients should receive high flow oxygen immediately if required

Oxygen is a drug and should always be prescribed unless you are in an emergency situation. Depending on local policies, oxygen may be prescribed on the paper drug chart, as a supplementary chart, or using an online 'ePrescribing' programme.

Most patients should have a SpO_2 target of 94% or higher. Patients at risk of CO_2 retention usually require a lower SpO_2 target, such as 88%–92%.

The arterial blood gas sample taken from this patient indicates that she has type 2 respiratory failure (low pO_2 and high pCO_2) with a chronic, compensated respiratory acidosis, as shown by the elevated bicarbonate level and the normal pH. She should, therefore, be prescribed oxygen aiming for a SpO_2 target of 88%–92%.

When prescribing oxygen, you should also indicate the device (e.g. Venturi mask, nasal cannulae, reservoir mask) and flow rate that should be used to deliver the oxygen. This should be reviewed each time your patient's oxygen requirement rises or falls.

History

A 48-year-old man presented to the emergency department complaining of chest pain. The pain was located over the centre of his chest and radiated to his left arm and up to his jaw. The pain was crushing in nature and the patient rated it as 10/10 in severity. There was associated nausea but no vomiting. The patient's past medical history included hypertension and type-2 diabetes mellitus. His regular medications were metformin 1 g BD and ramipril 5 mg OD; he had no known drug allergies.

The patient received a single dose of aspirin 300 mg PO and two sprays of GTN from the paramedics.

Examination

The patient appeared uncomfortable and diaphoretic but systems examination was unremarkable. His observations were as follows: temperature 37.0°C, HR 90 bpm, BP 150/90 mmHg, RR 18, and SpO_2 99% on room air.

Results

ECG: normal sinus rhythm; no ischaemic changes

Question

Which two of the following drugs should be prescribed next?

Morphine sulphate immediate release solution, 5–10 mg PO	☐
Morphine sulphate modified release solution 10 mg PO	☐
Morphine sulphate 10 mg IV	☐
Morphine sulphate 10 mg SC	☐
Clopidogrel 75 mg PO	☐
Clopidogrel 300 mg PO	☐

ANSWER

Morphine sulphate immediate release solution, 5–10 mg PO	☐
Morphine sulphate modified release solution 10 mg PO	☐
Morphine sulphate 10 mg IV	X
Morphine sulphate 10 mg SC	☐
Clopidogrel 75 mg PO	☐
Clopidogrel 300 mg PO	X

This patient has presented with acute chest pain and should be treated for possible acute coronary syndrome. As the patient is haemodynamically stable, the first step is to control his pain. Chest pain should be treated with sublingual GTN initially (as was given by the paramedics in this case) and, if needed, an intravenous infusion of GTN can later be prescribed for ongoing chest pain. In the interim, intravenous morphine sulphate should be given upon arrival to the emergency department. Morphine delivered intravenously acts more rapidly than the oral or subcutaneous routes.

Acute coronary syndrome is typically managed with dual antiplatelet therapy. The patient has already received aspirin from the paramedics and he should, therefore, be given an alternative anti-platelet agent. Clopidogrel is commonly prescribed, although some centres may prescribe ticagrelor or prasugrel instead. Loading doses of anti-platelet therapies (aspirin 300 mg, clopidogrel 300 mg, ticagrelor 180 mg, and prasugrel 60 mg) should be given for the first dose to achieve adequate inhibition of platelet activation and aggregation.

Other medications that could be prescribed for the patient once the above therapies have been given include an anti-emetic on the 'as required' side of the drug chart, as morphine can induce nausea in some patients, and oxygen if the patient develops hypoxia.

History

A 35-year-old man presented to hospital complaining of shortness of breath and a cough. The patient described worsening dyspnoea over the course of 3–4 weeks, with a non-productive cough and intermittent fevers. The patient's past medical history included HIV infection. He had no known drug allergies and was taking no regular medications, although he had been advised to take anti-retroviral therapy for several years. He worked as a bartender, smoked 5–10 cigarettes daily and drank 15–20 units of alcohol per week.

Examination

The patient appeared clinically well. He had coarse crackles over the right base and left mid-zone. His respiratory rate was 22 and his SpO_2 was 95% on room air, falling to 88% when mobilising.

Results

A chest X-ray showed bilateral perihilar consolidation and fine, reticular interstitial changes.

Sputum cultures: positive for *Pneumocystis jirovecii* pneumonia

Question

The patient has been diagnosed with *Pneumocystis jirovecii* pneumonia. He weighs 70 kg. Prescribe an appropriate course of oral antibiotics to treat this patient using the chart below.

DRUG (print approved name)		Dose	Date					
			6					
			8					
Signature	Date	Route	12					
Print name	Bleep	Pharmacy	14					
			18					
Additional information			22					

ANSWER

DRUG (print approved name)		Dose	Date						
			6						
CO-TRIMOXAZOLE		4.2 grams	(8)						
Signature	Date	Route	12						
a DOCTOR	01/01/2020	PO							
Print name	Bleep	Pharmacy	14						
A DOCTOR	1234		(18)						
Additional information			22						
To treat *Pneumocystis jirovecii* infection, 14 days									

The first-line treatment for *Pneumocystis jirovecii* (formerly known as *Pneumocystis carinii*) pneumonia is co-trimoxazole. This drug is a combination of sulfamethoxazole and trimethoprim.

The drug can be prescribed as an intravenous infusion or orally, at a dose of 120 mg/kg daily in 2–4 divided doses for 14–21 days. In a 70 kg patient, this is a total daily dose of 8400 mg or 8.4 g. In divided doses, this equates to 2.1 g QDS, 2.8 g TDS or 4.2 g BD.

History

A 26-year-old woman presented to hospital with fevers and vomiting. She reported a 4-day history of dysuria and urinary frequency and had developed right-sided abdominal pain over the preceding 24 h. She had no significant past medical history and took no regular medications. She worked as an art teacher, did not drink alcohol and had never smoked. She reported that she had recently started a new relationship and had several episodes of unprotected sexual intercourse over the past fortnight.

Examination

The patient had a temperature of 39.0°C. Her heart rate was 110 bpm and her blood pressure was 110/78 mmHg. Her abdomen was soft throughout but tender over the right flank.

Results

Urine dip: no blood, 2+ leucocytes, no protein, positive for nitrites, β-HCG negative

Preliminary urine culture result: Gram negative bacilli present

Question

The patient was treated for presumed pyelonephritis with intravenous gentamicin. Due to a prescribing error, she received two doses of gentamicin within an hour. An incident report form completed. Which four adverse effects are most likely to occur as a result of gentamicin toxicity?

Increased bruising	☐
Impaired liver function	☐
Impaired renal function	☐
Joint swelling	☐
Tendinopathy	☐
Tinnitus	☐
Vertigo	☐
Vomiting	☐

ANSWER

Increased bruising	☐
Impaired liver function	☐
Impaired renal function	X
Joint swelling	☐
Tendinopathy	☐
Tinnitus	X
Vertigo	X
Vomiting	X

Aminoglycosides are associated with a multitude of adverse effects. Vestibular ototoxicity is particularly well-recognised, with patients reporting symptoms of spontaneous episodic vertigo and potentially developing longstanding gait imbalance disorders. Patients may also develop tinnitus and hearing loss.

Aminoglycosides can also cause nephrotoxicity by altering phospholipid metabolism within the renal proximal tubular cells, and by additionally causing renal vasoconstriction. Reduced doses of aminoglycosides are typically prescribed for patients with pre-existing renal impairment.

Nausea, vomiting and skin reactions are also among the more commonly recognised adverse effects associated with aminoglycosides.

History

A 38-year-old woman presented to hospital complaining of right leg swelling and pain. She noticed the swelling develop approximately 24 h earlier and the right calf had since become increasingly tender. She was now struggling to weight-bear on her right leg. She denied any shortness of breath, cough or chest pain. She was 32-weeks pregnant and, until this point, the pregnancy has been uncomplicated. This was her third pregnancy and there were no significant complications associated with the previous two pregnancies. She had no past medical history and took no regular medications. She lived with her partner and children and did not work.

Examination

On examination, the right calf was erythematous and hot to touch. The diameter of the right calf was 10 cm greater than the diameter of the left calf. The pedal pulses were palpable bilaterally and sensation was intact throughout. Systemic examination was otherwise unremarkable.

Results

Bloods: WCC 7.2, Hb 112, MCV 83, Plt 289, Na 140, K 4.0, Creat 36

A Doppler ultrasound scan identified a right lower limb deep vein thrombosis extending into the popliteal vein.

Question

This patient has a confirmed deep vein thrombosis in her right leg. You have been advised by the haematology team to commence treatment with dalteparin. Please prescribe a regular prescription for this below. Her booking pregnancy weight was 62 kg.

DRUG (print approved name)		Dose	Date						
			6						
			8						
Signature	Date	Route	12						
Print name	Bleep	Pharmacy	14						
			18						
Additional information			22						

ANSWER

You should prescribe 12,500 units of dalteparin to be given subcutaneously, once daily. The correct prescription in this situation would therefore be:

DRUG (print approved name)		Dose	Date						
DALTEPARIN		12,500 UNITS	6						
			8						
Signature	Date	Route	12						
A Doctor	01/01/2020	SC							
Print name	Bleep	Pharmacy	14						
A DOCTOR	1234								
Additional information			(18)						
			22						

Current guidance for treating non-life threatening, non-recurring venous thromboembolism in pregnant patients is to prescribe subcutaneous low-molecular weight heparin, with dalteparin being a commonly used option. Please be aware that this is a higher dose of low molecular weight heparin than that used for venous thromboembolism prophylaxis.

In pregnant patients, their pre-pregnancy or booking weight should be used to guide the dosing of low-molecular weight heparin, rather than their weight during pregnancy, to prevent inappropriately high doses being given.

Some hospitals may have local guidance that advises individually tailored regimes, such as 'dalteparin dosed at 200 units per kg, rounded up to the nearest 500 units', but the British National Formulary and the majority of hospitals use the following weight brackets to guide treatment:

Weight	Treatment dose dalteparin
<46 kg	7,500 units OD
46–56 kg	10,000 units OD
57–68 kg	12,500 units OD
69–82 kg	15,000 units OD
83–100 kg	18,000 units OD
>100 kg	Discuss with on-call haematology team

CASE 34: PRESCRIBING 5

History
A 72-year-old woman presented to her general practitioner after experiencing muscle cramps on multiple occasions over the preceding weeks. She described developing cramps in her calf muscles and occasionally in her feet. The cramping pains had no clear precipitating factors, such as exercise or lying flat, and could come on at any point in the day or night. Her past medical history included hypertension and type-2 diabetes mellitus. Her regular medications were metformin 500 mg BD, lercanidipine 20 mg OD, and she had also commenced modified-release indapamide 1.5 mg OD 4 weeks earlier. She lived with her husband and was independent.

Examination
Systems examination was unremarkable – the patient appeared euvolaemic and her heart rate and blood pressure were within the normal range.

Results
Bloods: WCC 5.0, Hb 116, Plt 334, Na 137, K 2.5, Creat 60

ECG: normal sinus rhythm. No ST or T-wave abnormalities. U waves not present.

Question
The general practitioner diagnosed drug-induced hypokalaemia and advised that the patient attend the emergency department for treatment of this. Using the chart below, please prescribe an appropriate treatment for this patient's hypokalaemia.

INTRAVENOUS AND SUBCUTANEOUS INFUSIONS													
PRESCRIPTION								ADMINISTRATION					
Date	Route	Infusion fluid	Total vol (mls)	Additives	Dose	Rate/ duration	Prescriber (name/ signature)	Batch no.	Date & start time	Started by	Checked by	Time ended	Pharmacy

ANSWER

INTRAVENOUS AND SUBCUTANEOUS INFUSIONS												
PRESCRIPTION								ADMINISTRATION				
Date	Route	Infusion fluid	Total vol (mls)	Additives	Dose	Rate/ duration	Prescriber (name/ signature)	Batch no.	Date & start time	Started by	Checked by	Time ended	Pharmacy
01/01 /20	IV	0.9% NaCl	1000 mls	KCl	40 mmol	4 hours	*A Doctor*					

The patient has recently started taking the thiazide-like diuretic, indapamide, and has now developed hypokalaemia.

Patients with a potassium level of <3.0 mmol/L will need intravenous potassium replacement. Potassium can be administered in 5% glucose or 0.9% sodium chloride, with the latter being the most common option.

Between 20 and 40 mmol potassium chloride is usually prescribed in 1 L of fluid. The rate of administration can vary – in a ward-based setting, however, no more than 10 mmol of potassium chloride should be given per hour in order to reduce the risk of cardiac arrhythmias developing.

Concentrated preparations of potassium chloride can be given to patients who appear hypervolaemic to avoid overfilling them. Additionally, patients with severe hypokalaemia (<2.0 mmol/L) will need concentrated preparations of potassium chloride that can be administered more rapidly than 10 mmol/h. These patients should all be managed in a critical care unit setting where appropriate vascular access and cardiac monitoring will be available.

It is also worth noting that any patient with hypokalaemia should also have their serum magnesium levels checked. This is because hypomagnesaemia may lead to refractory hypokalaemia by inhibiting ATP-dependent potassium channels and increasing potassium secretion. If hypomagnesaemia is present, magnesium and potassium will need to be replaced simultaneously.

In this case, the patient has a moderate hypokalaemia and should be prescribed 40 mmol potassium chloride in 1 L of intravenous 0.9% sodium chloride. The rate of fluid administration will depend on the fluid status of the patient – she currently appears euvolaemic and has no past medical history suggestive of heart failure and you can therefore prescribe the fluid to run over 4 h (although prescriptions of 6–8 h would also be correct). She should have her potassium level checked again once the infusion is completed.

History

A 19-year-old woman presented to hospital complaining of shortness of breath and cough. She had been feeling unwell with increasing difficulty in breathing over the preceding 6 h. She had been otherwise well recently, aside from a wrist injury that she sustained 24 h ago playing badminton. She had managed this with ice packs and simple analgesia. Her past medical history was significant for asthma. She had no known drug allergies and her only medication was a salbutamol inhaler that was used 'as needed'. The patient was studying philosophy at university, did not smoke, and drank approximately 14 units of alcohol per week.

Examination

On examination, the patient was visibly dyspnoeic. There was a widespread polyphonic expiratory wheeze heard throughout her chest. Her respiratory rate was 20 breaths per minute and her peripheral oxygen saturations (SpO_2) were 100% on room air.

Results

Chest X-ray: clear lung fields, no signs of consolidation or collapse

Questions

1. Which three medications below should be initially prescribed for the patient in the emergency department?
2. Which one medication is most likely to have precipitated the onset of the patient's symptoms?

			1	2
Beclomethasone	200 μg	INH	☐	☐
Hydrocortisone	200 mg	IV	☐	☐
Ibuprofen	400 mg	PO	☐	☐
Ipratropium bromide	500 μg	NEB	☐	☐
Paracetamol	1 g	PO	☐	☐
Prednisolone	40 mg	PO	☐	☐
Salbutamol	2 puffs	INH	☐	☐
Salbutamol	2.5 mg	NEB	☐	☐

ANSWERS

			1	2
Beclomethasone	200 µg	INH	☐	☐
Hydrocortisone	200 mg	IV	X	☐
Ibuprofen	400 mg	PO	☐	X
Ipratropium bromide	500 µg	NEB	X	☐
Paracetamol	1 g	PO	☐	☐
Prednisolone	40 mg	PO	☐	☐
Salbutamol	2 puffs	INH	☐	☐
Salbutamol	2.5 mg	NEB	X	☐

1. In the initial phase of management, the patient should be treated with the β2 adrenergic agonist, salbutamol. This medication induces bronchodilation by causing relaxation of the smooth muscles surrounding the airways. The nebulised route of administration is a more effective way of delivering salbutamol than via inhalers.

   Nebulised ipratropium bromide should also be prescribed. This is an antimuscarinic agent that acts on airway muscarinic receptors to reduce airway smooth muscle contraction, thus inducing bronchodilation.

   Lastly, a corticosteroid should be prescribed. Steroids act to suppress the immune response and thus reduce inflammation of the airways. Intravenous therapy is generally considered to be preferable, although it is not clear that this is more efficacious than the oral route of administration in patients who can take medications by mouth. Intravenous hydrocortisone is commonly used to treat acute exacerbations of asthma.

2. Drugs that can trigger bronchoconstriction, including beta blockers, adenosine, and non-steroidal anti-inflammatory drugs (NSAIDs) should be avoided, where possible, in patients with asthma. This patient recently sustained a wrist injury and has been self-medicating with simple analgesia. Ibuprofen is an NSAID, and drugs in this class can trigger wheeze in up to 20% of patients with asthma.

History

A 60-year-old woman was admitted to hospital with fever and rigors. She described a 3-day history of worsening dysuria and left flank pain. She reported feeling intermittently hot and cold with several episodes of shaking uncontrollably. She felt nauseated and had vomited twice. Her past medical history included depression and osteoarthritis. She took no regular medications. She worked as a dance instructor and lived with her partner.

Examination

On examination, the patient was febrile with a temperature of 38.2°C. Her heart sounds were normal and her chest was clear. Her abdomen was soft with mild left iliac fossa and left flank tenderness.

Results

Urine dip: 2+ leucocytes, 1+ erythrocytes, positive for nitrites

Bloods: WCC 17.3, Hb 120, Plt 412, Na 135, K 4.1, Creat 55, CRP 129

Question

You are asked to prescribe an intravenous infusion of gentamicin for this patient. The patient weighs 60 kg and has a body mass index (BMI) of 22.

ONCE ONLY MEDICATIONS									
Date	Medication	Dose	Route	Time of dose	Signature	Prescriber	Given by	Time given	Pharmacy

ANSWER

ONCE ONLY MEDICATIONS									
Date	Medication	Dose	Route	Time of dose	Signature	Prescriber	Given by	Time given	Pharmacy
01/01/20	GENTAMICIN	420 mg	IV	12:00	*A Doctor*	A DOCTOR			

The patient is likely to have pyelonephritis and should be treated with an intravenous infusion of gentamicin. The British National Formulary recommends a dose of 5–7 mg/kg in an adult patient with normal renal function. Local antibiotic guidelines may vary, and some recommend a reduced dose (e.g. 3 mg/kg) in elderly patients or those with reduced creatinine clearance. For patients who are significantly overweight, ideal body weight should be used to calculate the appropriate dose.

In this case, a dose of 300–420 mg should be prescribed intravenously as soon as possible, following a diagnosis of pyelonephritis. Serum gentamicin levels can be taken post-dose to monitor clearance of the drug and to guide repeat dosing.

History

A 22-year-old man was admitted to the intensive care unit with bacterial meningitis. He was treated with intravenous antibiotics and was later intubated and ventilated to protect his airway. As he was likely to be unable to eat a normal diet for several days, the nutrition team advised that he be fed enterally via a nasogastric tube to optimise his nutritional status.

Question

The nutrition team have recommended that the patient commence standard 1 kcal/mL enteral feed at a rate of 30 mL/kg/day. The patient weighs 72 kg and the feed will be run continuously over 24 h. Please calculate the rate at which the enteral feed should run. You can use a calculator if needed.

The enteral feed should run at ☐ mL/min.

ANSWER

The patient weighs 72 kg and requires 30 mL/kg per day: $72 \times 30 = 2160$ mL/day.

2160 mL per day is equivalent to 90 mL/h, which is equivalent to 1.5 mL/min.

History

A 16-year-old man was brought to hospital after developing acute confusion. His mother reported that he was unsure of where he was or who his family were upon waking this morning and that he had complained of fever and cough over the past 2 days. He had no past medical history, took no regular medications and had no unwell contacts. He was a college student and lived with his family.

Examination

On examination, he was agitated and confused. He was not orientated to time or place. There was a vesicular rash over his torso and upper limbs.

Results

CT head: no acute pathology

Question

The emergency department consultant is concerned that the patient could have varicella zoster encephalitis and asks you to prescribe regular treatment for this on the chart below. The patient weighs 70 kg.

DRUG (print approved name)		Dose	Date					
			6					
			8					
Signature	Date	Route	12					
Print name	Bleep	Pharmacy	14					
			18					
Additional information			22					

ANSWER

DRUG (print approved name)		Dose	Date					
ACICLOVIR		700 mg	6					
			(8)					
Signature	Date	Route	12					
A Doctor	01/01/20	IV						
Print name	Bleep	Pharmacy	(14)					
A DOCTOR	1234							
			18					
Additional information			(22)					
10–14 days duration, for suspected viral encephalitis								

The patient should be prescribed an anti-viral treatment. Aciclovir is commonly used in many hospitals to treat suspected viral encephalitis. The recommended dose for suspected herpes zoster or varicella zoster encephalitis is 10 mg/kg every 8 h, given for 10–14 days. The correct prescription is shown above.

CASE 39: PRESCRIBING 8

History

A 45-year-old woman was brought to hospital after developing shortness of breath. She reported that she had recently started taking a course of flucloxacillin 500 mg PO QDS for an infected cut on her finger. She took the second dose of the antibiotic and developed shortness of breath and chest tightness approximately 20 min later. She had no past medical history, took no regular medications and had no known allergies. She worked as a university lecturer, drank 20 units of alcohol per week and was an ex-smoker.

Examination

On examination, the patient had a visibly swollen tongue but was able to speak. Her respiratory rate was 36 and there was an audible wheeze throughout her chest; oxygen saturations were 100% on 15 L O$_2$ via a non-rebreathe bag. Her heart rate was 130 bpm and her blood pressure was 80/50 mmHg.

Question

Prescribe one drug that should be given immediately in this scenario.

PATIENT DETAILS (affix sticker)	
Given name	ANNA
Family name	PATIENT
Patient ID	123456A
DOB	01/01/1970
Sex	M ☐ F ☒

ALLERGIES AND ADVERSE REACTIONS

☒ Nil known   ☐ Unknown

A DOCTOR Signature   01/01/20 Date

Drug (or other)	Reaction

ONCE ONLY MEDICATIONS

Date	Medication	Route	Dose	Time of dose	Signature	Prescriber	Given by	Time given	Pharmacy

ANSWER

PATIENT DETAILS (affix sticker)	
Given name	ANNA
Family name	PATIENT
Patient ID	123456A
DOB	01/01/1970
Sex	M ☐ F ☒

ALLERGIES AND ADVERSE REACTIONS

☐ Nil known   ☐ Unknown

A DOCTOR Signature   01/01/20 Date

Drug (or other)	Reaction
PENICILLINS	ANAPHYLAXIS

ONCE ONLY MEDICATIONS

Date	Medication	Dose	Route	Time of dose	Signature	Prescriber	Given by	Time given	Pharmacy
01/01/20	ADRENALINE 1:1,000	0.5 mg	IM	12:00	*A DOCTOR*	A DOCTOR			
01/01/20	CHLORPHENAMINE	10 mg	IV	12:00	*A DOCTOR*	A DOCTOR			
01/01/20	HYDROCORTISONE	200 mg	IV	12:00	*A DOCTOR*	A DOCTOR			

Assuming that the patient is still conscious with an intact airway, the most important drug to administer at this point is adrenaline intramuscularly at a dose of 0.5 mg (0.5 mL of adrenaline 1 mg/mL [1:1000]).

Although not part of the question, there are other changes that would need to be made to the drug chart if this were a real-life scenario. First, on the infusion side of the drug chart, 1 L of 0.9% sodium chloride or another crystalloid fluid should be prescribed to run over 15 min. The antihistamine, chlorphenamine (10 mg IM or IV), corticosteroid, and hydrocortisone (200 mg IM or IV) should also be given – they have a slow onset of action but may be of benefit in some patients. The antihistamine may reduce histamine-mediated bronchoconstriction and vasodilation, whilst the steroid can reduce and lessen the duration of the inflammatory response.

Lastly, the patient's drug chart should be amended to state that she is allergic to penicillin-based drugs. If there is any doubt as to the cause of reaction, then formal allergy testing can be performed at a later date.

History

A 52-year-old woman was admitted to hospital with a 5-day history of worsening shortness of breath, cough and right-sided chest pain. She had no significant past medical history and took no regular medications.

Examination

The patient was febrile at 38.2°C. Her heart rate was 100 bpm, her blood pressure was 120/80 mmHg and her heart sounds were dual with no murmurs. There were crackles at her right lung base and her oxygen saturations were 90% on room air.

Results

Bloods: WCC 13.4, Hb 138, Plt 375, Na 139, K 4.1, Creat 54, CRP 87

Chest X-ray: consolidation over the right lower zone

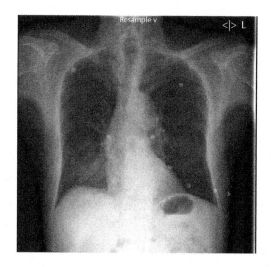

Question

Intravenous antibiotics were commenced and the patient was advised that she was likely to be admitted to hospital for at least 48 h. The patient weighs 60 kg. You are asked to prescribe pharmacological venous thromboembolism (VTE) prophylaxis for her, using the form below:

		Date						
DRUG (print approved name)	**Dose**	6						
CO-AMOXICLAV	1.2 g	⑧						
Signature **Date** **Route**		12						
A Doctor 01/01/20 IV								
Print name **Bleep** **Pharmacy**		⑭						
A DOCTOR 1234		18						
Additional information								
5 day course, community-acquired pneumonia		㉒						
DRUG (print approved name)	**Dose**	6						
		8						
Signature **Date** **Route**		12						
		14						
Print name **Bleep** **Pharmacy**								
		18						
Additional information		22						

ANSWER

DRUG (print approved name)		Dose	Date							
			6							
CO-AMOXICLAV		1.2 g	⑧							
Signature	Date	Route	12							
A Doctor	01/01/20	IV								
Print name	Bleep	Pharmacy	⑭							
A DOCTOR	1234		18							
Additional information			㉒							
5 day course, community-acquired pneumonia										
DRUG (print approved name)		Dose	6							
			8							
DALTEPARIN		5000 UNITS								
Signature	Date	Route	12							
A Doctor	01/01/20	SC								
Print name	Bleep	Pharmacy	14							
A DOCTOR	1234		⑱							
Additional information			22							

Unwell medical patients who are likely to spend 24 h or more in hospital should be offered VTE prophylaxis. The first-line option for VTE prophylaxis is low molecular weight heparin (LMWH) and local guidelines will vary as to which LMWH is routinely prescribed. Doses of LMWH vary based on the patient's weight and renal function. Patients with impaired renal function may be prescribed unfractionated heparin instead of LMWH.

Potential options for VTE prophylaxis with LMWH include dalteparin 5000 units OD or enoxaparin 40 mg OD.

Question

Of the cardiovascular drugs below, identify the *two* that have dosage errors:

Amlodipine	10 mg	PO	OD	☐
Bendroflumethiazide	25 mg	PO	OD	☐
Bisoprolol	5 mg	PO	OD	☐
Candesartan	8 mg	PO	OD	☐
Digoxin	125 mg	PO	OD	☐
Doxazosin	8 mg	PO	BD	☐
Ramipril	5 mg	PO	OD	☐

ANSWER

Amlodipine	10 mg	PO	OD	☐
Bendroflumethiazide	25 mg	PO	OD	X
Bisoprolol	5 mg	PO	OD	☐
Candesartan	8 mg	PO	OD	☐
Digoxin	125 mg	PO	OD	X
Doxazosin	8 mg	PO	BD	☐
Ramipril	5 mg	PO	OD	☐

Bendroflumethiazide is prescribed at a dose of 2.5 mg OD for hypertension, but may be prescribed at higher doses of up to 10 mg OD.

Digoxin is typically prescribed at doses of 62.5 up to 250 micrograms (not milligrams) orally for the management of atrial fibrillation or atrial flutter, or for heart failure. It is important to ensure that you prescribe the correct units to prevent catastrophic dosing errors.

History
A 50-year-old man was admitted to hospital with a painful right leg. He had been feeling feverish and generally unwell for the past 3 days. His past medical history included pulmonary tuberculosis and a recent hospital admission with pneumonia. He was not taking any regular medications. He had no fixed abode and usually slept on the streets. He drank approximately 30 units of alcohol per week and smoked 20 cigarettes daily.

Examination
On examination, he was noted to be febrile and to have a hot, swollen, erythematous right leg.

Progress
The patient was diagnosed with a right lower limb cellulitis. Whilst he was in hospital, he was additionally noted to have an erythematous rash between the web spaces of his fingers and toes and across his wrists bilaterally.

Question
Prescribe appropriate topical therapy to treat the patient's scabies infestation.

ONCE ONLY MEDICATIONS									
Date	Medication	Dose	Route	Time of dose	Signature	Prescriber	Given by	Time given	Pharmacy

ANSWER

ONCE ONLY MEDICATIONS									
Date	Medication	Dose	Route	Time of dose	Signature	Prescriber	Given by	Time given	Pharmacy
01/01/20	PERMETHRIN 5%	1 APPLICATION	TOP	13:00	*A Doctor*	A DOCTOR			

This patient is infested with the skin mite, *Sarcoptes scabiei*. The standard treatment of scabies infestations consists of a weekly topical application of permethrin. This is a pyrethroid medication that paralyses insects by preventing axonal repolarisation.

Patients should apply permethrin topically, aiming to cover the whole body (including the face and hands) in a layer of the liquid or cream. This should be washed off after 8–12 h. The treatment should be repeated 1 week later, and the patient must avoid exposing themselves to clothes, bedding, or towels that may have retained scabies mites.

Crusted scabies, also known as Norwegian scabies, is a severe form of scabies infestation that occurs in patients who are immunocompromised or very frail. In these cases, the *Sarcoptes scabiei* mites should be treated with both topical permethrin and oral ivermectin (a macrocyclic lactone insecticide).

History

A 57-year-old woman was admitted to hospital with nausea and vomiting. She described a 2-day history of frequent episodes of vomiting with several episodes of watery brown diarrhoea. She was initially vomiting food matter but had since been vomiting bilious fluid up to twice per hour; there had been no blood in her vomitus or stool. Her past medical history included type 2 diabetes mellitus, hypertension and osteoarthritis of the left hip. Her regular medications are listed below. She worked as a recruitment supervisor, had never smoked and did not drink alcohol.

Results

Bloods: WCC 12.1, Hb 128, Plt 451, Na 136, K 3.4, Creat 174 (baseline 56 µmol/L 3 months earlier), CRP 45

Question

Which *four* of the patient's regular medications listed below should be withheld in view of her blood results?

Amlodipine	5 mg	PO	OD	☐
Bendroflumethiazide	2.5 mg	PO	OD	☐
Ibuprofen	400 mg	PO	TDS	☐
Metformin	500 mg	PO	OD	☐
Omeprazole	20 mg	PO	OD	☐
Paracetamol	1 g	PO	QDS	☐
Ramipril	5 mg	PO	OD	☐
Ranitidine	150 mg	PO	BD	☐

ANSWER

Amlodipine	5 mg	PO	OD	☐
Bendroflumethiazide	2.5 mg	PO	OD	X
Ibuprofen	400 mg	PO	TDS	X
Metformin	500 mg	PO	OD	X
Omeprazole	20 mg	PO	OD	☐
Paracetamol	1 g	PO	QDS	☐
Ramipril	5 mg	PO	OD	X
Ranitidine	150 mg	PO	BD	☐

The patient's blood results show that she has an acute kidney injury, likely secondary to the symptoms of gastroenteritis that she has reported. She should be treated with intravenous fluids and her fluid balance status should be closely monitored. Repeat bloods should be taken 8–12 h later to ensure that her renal function is improving.

During an episode of acute kidney injury, patients should have their regular medications reviewed to avoid administering: (i) non-essential medications that could contribute to their poor renal function (i.e. nephrotoxic drugs) or (ii) medications that may not be adequately cleared and could thus cause signs and symptoms of toxicity to develop.

This patient is taking the diuretic, bendroflumethiazide, which will further contribute to her dehydration; and the ACE inhibitor, ramipril, which will reduce glomerular pressure and may also cause hyperkalaemia. Partial metabolism of ramirpril occurs in the renal system and 60% of the drug is eliminated via the urine. Metformin is eliminated almost entirely via the renal system and metformin concentrations can accumulate in impaired renal function, resulting in a lactic acidosis developing. Ibuprofen, as with other non-steroidal anti-inflammatory drugs (NSAIDs), reduces renal blood flow by inhibiting prostaglandin synthesis.

Once the patient has recovered from the acute kidney injury, their medications should be reviewed once again, and those medications that were withheld may be re-introduced and uptitrated as appropriate.

History

A 76-year-old woman was brought to hospital after her daughter found her to be confused. Her daughter reported visiting daily and had noticed the patient becoming increasingly disorientated and drowsy over the past 2–3 days. The patient's past medical history included osteoporosis, a recent elective hip replacement, and diet-controlled type 2 diabetes mellitus. She was a retired history teacher, lived alone, and was independent until her surgery 2 weeks earlier. She did not drink alcohol and had never smoked.

Examination

The patient was drowsy but roused to voice (Glasgow Coma Scale 13 – E3, V4, M6). Her pupils were 1 mm bilaterally. Her heart rate was 45, her blood pressure was 100/70 mmHg, and her heart sounds were normal with no murmurs. Her respiratory rate was 10, her peripheral oxygen saturations (SpO$_2$) were 92% on room air, and her chest was clear. Her abdomen was soft and non-tender. The operation wound was healing well and appeared clean and dry with no signs of infection.

Results

Bloods: WCC 8.3, Hb 120, Plt 390, Na 137, K 4.5, Creat 50, CRP 35

Questions

1. From the medications listed below, please select three that may have contributed to her current condition.
2. Please select one medication that should be given to the patient immediately.

				1	2
Co-codamol 8/500	2 tablets	PO	QDS	☐	☐
Dihydrocodeine	30 mg	PO	QDS	☐	☐
Ibuprofen	400 mg	PO	TDS	☐	☐
Lidocaine 5% medicated plaster	One plaster	TOP	Once only	☐	☐
Morphine sulphate immediate release solution	5 mg	PO	4 hourly	☐	☐
Naloxone	100 µg	IV	Once only	☐	☐
Naproxen	250 mg	PO	QDS	☐	☐
Paracetamol	1 g	PO	QDS	☐	☐

ANSWERS

				1	2
Co-codamol 8/500	2 tablets	PO	QDS	X	☐
Dihydrocodeine	30 mg	PO	QDS	X	☐
Ibuprofen	400 mg	PO	TDS	☐	☐
Lidocaine 5% medicated plaster	One plaster	TOP	Once only	☐	☐
Morphine sulphate immediate release solution	5 mg	PO	4 hourly	X	☐
Naloxone	100 µg	IV	Once only	☐	X
Naproxen	250 mg	PO	QDS	☐	☐
Paracetamol	1 g	PO	QDS	☐	☐

1. The patient has clear signs of opioid toxicity – she is drowsy and confused, has pin-point pupils, a reduced respiratory rate, and has low oxygen saturations indicative of respiratory depression. The opioid medications, dihydrocodeine and morphine sulphate, should therefore be stopped.

   Co-codamol is a combination therapy containing codeine phosphate and paracetamol and should also be stopped. Combination medications are often overlooked when reviewing medications and it is common for medications containing paracetamol to be prescribed alongside paracetamol, thus resulting in an overdose. In the hospital setting, it is preferable to prescribe the constituent medications separately to avoid dosing errors.

2. Naloxone is an opiod receptor antagonist and should be administered in this case to reverse the effects of opioid toxicity. As the patient is still awake and stable from a haemodynamic and respiratory perspective, a low dose of naloxone (e.g. 50–100 µg) should be administered initially, to rouse the patient without suddenly reversing the analgesic effects of the opioids that she has been taking.

   In emergency situations (loss of consciousness, severe respiratory depression, respiratory arrest, or haemodynamic compromise), naloxone should be administered in 400 µg boluses, up to a total dose of 2 mg – if the patient has not responded to 2 mg naloxone, then the diagnosis of opioid toxicity should be reviewed.

CASE 45: PLANNING MANAGEMENT 4

History
A 69-year-old man was presented to hospital complaining of a 6-h history of abdominal pain and several episodes of vomiting small amounts (approximately one tablespoon on each occasion) of blood. The patient denied any fevers or recent illnesses and did not report any change to his bowel motions. His past medical history included previous peptic ulcer disease, ischaemic heart disease, and osteoarthritis. He had no known drug allergies. He was a retired teacher who lived with his partner, smoked 10 cigarettes per day, and drank 15–20 units of alcohol per week.

Examination
On examination, the patient had epigastric abdominal pain on deep palpation and a digital rectal examination identified tarry black stool, consistent with melaena. The patient's heart rate was 90 bpm and his blood pressure was 110/70 mmHg.

Results
Bloods: WCC 9.2, Hb 108, MCV 80, Plt 405, Na 137, K 3.9, urea 12.2, Creat 70, INR 1.0

Questions
1. Which *three* of the patient's regular medications should be withheld?
2. Which *one* medication should be commenced?

				1	2
Aspirin	75 mg	PO	OD	☐	☐
Alendronic acid	10 mg	PO	OD	☐	☐
Calcium/vitamin D supplements	2 tablets	PO	OD	☐	☐
Ibuprofen	200 mg	PO	TDS	☐	☐
Omeprazole	40 mg	PO	OD	☐	☐
Pantoprazole	40 mg	IV	OD	☐	☐
Paracetamol	1 g	PO	QDS	☐	☐
Ranitidine	150 mg	PO	BD	☐	☐

ANSWERS

				1	2
Aspirin	75 mg	PO	OD	X	☐
Alendronic acid	10 mg	PO	OD	X	☐
Calcium/vitamin D supplements	2 tablets	PO	OD	☐	☐
Ibuprofen	200 mg	PO	TDS	X	☐
Omeprazole	40 mg	PO	OD	☐	☐
Pantoprazole	40 mg	IV	OD	☐	X
Paracetamol	1 g	PO	QDS	☐	☐
Ranitidine	150 mg	PO	BD	☐	☐

1. The patient is likely to be kept 'nil-by-mouth' for 24 h in case an emergency oesophago-gastro-duodenoscopy (OGD) is required, but regular medications are usually given, if needed, to patients who remain haemodynamically stable.

   Both aspirin and ibuprofen are non-steroidal anti-inflammatory drugs (NSAIDs). These drugs inhibit the COX enzymes and subsequently inhibit prostaglandin synthesis. Prostaglandins have a protective effect on the gastric mucosa and reduce the risk of gastrointestinal ulceration. Aspirin is also anti-platelet agent and thus will impair platelet activation and aggregation, and subsequent clot formation. This should be held as it will increase the risk of bleeding.

   Alendronic acid is a bisphosphonate that can cause local irritation of the oesophagus and gastric mucosa if not consumed correctly (with a full glass of water, whilst sitting upright or standing for 30–60 min following this). This medication should be withheld whilst there is a possible upper gastrointestinal bleed.

2. The patient should be prescribed intravenous pantoprazole. In the context of an acute upper gastrointestinal bleed, a high-dose intravenous infusion of an antisecretory therapy, usually a proton-pump inhibitor, should be commenced. This is commonly either pantoprazole or omeprazole and is given as a bolus. Over the next 24 h, a continuous intravenous infusion of a proton-pump inhibitor may be prescribed (e.g. pantoprazole 8 mg/h) or, alternatively, daily intravenous boluses can be administered depending on the local policy.

History

A 54-year-old man underwent a right hemicolectomy to treat adenocarcinoma of the bowel. Two days later, he developed acute left-sided chest pain that was exacerbated by coughing and deep inspiration.

Examination

The patient was awake and alert. His heart rate was 100 bpm and his blood pressure was 140/90 mmHg. His heart sounds were normal. His chest was clear and his peripheral oxygen saturations (SpO_2) were 96% on room air. There was no peripheral oedema. The patient had a swollen, erythematous left calf, clinically in keeping with a deep vein thrombosis.

Results

Bloods: Troponin T 5 (reference range <14 ng/L), NT pro-BNP 120

CT pulmonary angiogram: multiple bilateral subsegmental pulmonary emboli with no evidence of right heart strain

Question

The surgical team advised that the patient was still at significant risk of having a major post-operative bleed. From the management options below, please select the *one* most appropriate plan for this patient.

Commence a direct oral anticoagulant	☐
Commence an intravenous unfractionated heparin infusion	☐
Commence thrombolysis therapy	☐
Commence 'treatment dose' low molecular weight heparin	☐
Do not treat the pulmonary emboli as the patient is at risk of bleeding	☐

ANSWER

Commence a direct oral anticoagulant	☐
Commence an intravenous unfractionated heparin infusion	X
Commence thrombolysis therapy	☐
Commence 'treatment dose' low molecular weight heparin	☐
Do not treat the pulmonary emboli as the patient is at risk of bleeding	☐

This patient has several pulmonary emboli and these should be treated to prevent further clot extension. The patient is haemodynamically stable with no evidence of cardiac compromise (troponin T and NT pro-BNP levels are not elevated); so thrombolysis is therefore not indicated.

Unfractionated heparin has a half-life of 1–2 h, whereas low molecular weight heparins generally have a longer half-life of 4–6 h. The direct oral anticoagulants have varying half-lives, from 5 to 14 h. Unfractionated heparin is therefore the safest option to use in this scenario as the infusion can be stopped if there are any signs of bleeding and the drug will then be rapidly cleared.

CASE 47: PROVIDING INFORMATION 1

History

A 35-year-old woman was reviewed by the haematology team in the outpatient department. She had been asked to attend due to difficulties in establishing an appropriate dose of warfarin. The patient's past medical history included antiphospholipid syndrome that was diagnosed following several episodes of venous thrombolemboli developing. Her only regular prescribed medication was warfarin; her regular doses of this had varied from 2 to 8 mg OD. She worked as a yoga instructor and did not drink alcohol or smoke cigarettes.

Results

INR 1.5 (target INR 2.0–3.0)

Question

The patient's INR result has fluctuated considerably since initiating therapy. On direct questioning, she admits to taking a variety of over-the-counter and herbal remedies, listed below. Which *two* of the non-prescription treatments/supplements below will you advise that the patient should stop taking?

Chia seeds	☐
Cranberry juice	☐
Omega-3 fish oil	☐
Manuka honey	☐
St John's wort	☐

ANSWER

Chia seeds	☐
Cranberry juice	X
Omega-3 fish oil	☐
Manuka honey	☐
St John's wort	X

It is important to ask all patients whether they take any over-the-counter or herbal remedies, as these are often omitted from drug histories. Many herbal or plant-based supplements have significant interactions with prescription medications, altering their metabolism to either increase or reduce their efficacy. Unlicensed Ayurvedic and traditional Chinese medicines have been associated with cases of hepatotoxicity and nephrotoxicity and some samples have also been found to contain unsafe quantities of lead, mercury and arsenic.

The anticoagulant, warfarin, is metabolised by the cytochrome P_{450} system. Warfarin has a narrow therapeutic index and interacts with many other prescription medications and herbal or plant-based supplements. Both cranberry juice and St John's wort interact with the cytochrome P_{450} system and can affect the metabolism of warfarin. Cranberry juice increases the International Normalised Ratio (INR), whilst St John's wort decreases the INR through inhibition and induction of cytochrome P_{450} isoenzymes, respectively. Other herbal and plant-based supplements that may interact with warfarin include alfalfa, chamomile, garlic, ginger, ginseng, glucosamine, liquorice, turmeric and wormwood.

History

A 75-year-old female patient was admitted to hospital with diarrhoea and vomiting. Her bloods showed an acute kidney injury, but her serum electrolyte levels were within the reference ranges.

Question

You decide to prescribe intravenous fluids for the patient. You choose to administer 1000 mL Hartmann's solution (compound sodium lactate) using an infusion set that delivers 20 drops/mL. What rate should the drip be set at (to the nearest drop per minute) to allow the infusion to be completed over 8 h?

The drip rate should be ☐ drops per minute.

ANSWER

The infusion set delivers 20 drops/mL so there will be 20,000 drops in 1000 mL to be delivered over 8 h.

This is equivalent to 20,000 drops being delivered in 480 min, which works out as 41.67 drops/min.

The answer is 42 drops/min.

History

A 17-year-old man was admitted to hospital after developing a generalised vesicular rash over the preceding 24 h. He became acutely confused in the emergency department and was diagnosed with probable varicella zoster encephalitis.

Question

The patient has been prescribed a 10 mg/kg dose of aciclovir to be given as an intravenous infusion in the emergency department.

Vials of aciclovir powder are reconstituted in 0.9% sodium chloride.

You are asked to prepare a solution at a concentration of 25 mg aciclovir per mL and run it over 1 h.

The patient weighs 75 kg.

Please calculate the rate of the aciclovir infusion that will be delivered via a controlled-rate infusion pump.

The aciclovir infusion should run at ☐ mL/min.

100 Cases in Clinical Pharmacology, Therapeutics and Prescribing

ANSWER

The patient weighs 75 kg and requires a dose of 10 mg/kg aciclovir. He, therefore, requires 750 mg aciclovir.

The aciclovir is reconstituted to a concentration of 25 mg aciclovir per mL of 0.9% sodium chloride.

Therefore, 750 mg of aciclovir will require 30 mL of 0.9% sodium chloride. The patient should receive the 30 mL solution over 60 min and should thus receive 0.5 mL/min.

History

A 36-year-old woman was reviewed in the rheumatology clinic after developing a flare of her rheumatoid arthritis. She had experienced widespread joint swelling. She also complained of extreme fatigue and a feeling of general malaise. She had no other past medical history and usually managed her rheumatoid arthritis pain with naproxen tablets. She worked as a swimming instructor, did not drink alcohol and had never smoked.

Examination

There was obvious swelling of the small joints of her hands, her wrists, and her ankles and movement was limited by pain. Systems examination was otherwise unremarkable.

Question

The rheumatology consultant decided to prescribe corticosteroid therapy to suppress the inflammatory response. The patient asks whether there are any side effects associated with corticosteroids.

Please tick two adverse effects below that are commonly associated with corticosteroid use.

Alopecia	☐
Constipation	☐
Insomnia	☐
Urinary retention	☐
Weight gain	☐

ANSWER

Alopecia	☐
Constipation	☐
Insomnia	X
Urinary retention	☐
Weight gain	X

Corticosteroids are associated with a variety of adverse effects, including (but not limited to):

- Altered mental state, including anxiety, mood disorders, and psychosis
- Cushing's syndrome
- Hypertension
- Impaired wound healing
- Increased risk of infections, particularly including candidiasis
- Insomnia and other sleep disorders (including nightmares)
- Peptic ulcer disease
- Weight gain – due to both increased appetite and fluid retention

Patients taking corticosteroids steroids for a duration of several weeks will develop adrenal suppression where their body downregulates production of endogenous steroids such as cortisol and aldosterone in response to the exogenous steroids. Patients should thus be advised to gradually wean down their corticosteroids rather than suddenly stopping the course.

History

A 60-year-old man was asked to attend the emergency department following an abnormal routine blood test earlier that day. He had been feeling well recently; the blood test was taken following recent changes to his regular medications. His past medical history was significant for hypertension only. His current medications were ramipril 5 mg OD and spironolactone 25 mg OD. He worked as a retail manager, did not drink alcohol regularly and had never smoked.

Results

Bloods from the emergency department: WCC 10.2, Hb 150, Plt 327, Na 135, K 7.1, Creat 117, CRP <1

ECG: Normal sinus rhythm with tall 'tented' T waves across all leads

Question

Based on the above information, which *three* treatment options below would be most appropriate to commence immediately?

Actrapid 10 units in 50 mL glucose 50% IV	☐
Fixed rate intravenous insulin infusion 0.1 unit/kg/h	☐
Calcium gluconate 10% 10 mL IV	☐
Calcium resonium (polystyrene sulfonate) 15 g PO	☐
Salbutamol 250 µg IV	☐
Salbutamol 10 mg NEB	☐
Sodium bicarbonate 1 g PO	☐

ANSWER

Actrapid 10 units in 50 mL glucose 50% IV	X
Fixed rate intravenous insulin infusion 0.1 unit/kg/h	☐
Calcium gluconate 10% 10 mL IV	X
Calcium resonium (polystyrene sulfonate) 15 g PO	☐
Salbutamol 250 µg IV	☐
Salbutamol 10 mg NEB	X
Sodium bicarbonate 1 g PO	☐

Acute hyperkalaemia (serum potassium level ≥6.0 mmol/L) can be life-threatening and should be addressed urgently. The ECG shows tall T 'tented' waves consistent with hyperkalaemic changes.

Intravenous access should be established immediately and the patient should be given:

1. Calcium gluconate 10% 10 mL intravenously – this stabilises the cardiac myocyte cell membrane to reduce the risk of arrhythmias developing.
2. Actrapid 10 units in 50 mL glucose 50% IV – insulin stimulates the Na-K ATPase pump, which allows potassium to enter cells, and should be administered with glucose to prevent hypoglycaemia from developing. Patients who receive this therapy should have their blood glucose monitored over the next 6 h.
3. Salbutamol 10 mg NEB – salbutamol also stimulates the Na-K ATPase pump via β2 receptor stimulation, driving potassium intracellularly. There is some evidence that intravenous salbutamol can be effective in reducing hyperkalaemia; however, in a ward-based setting, nebulised salbutamol is safer.

Patients with a metabolic acidosis may benefit from sodium bicarbonate therapy; however, this is usually administered intravenously in the acute setting. Patients with refractory hyperkaelaemia or renal failure should be discussed with the renal or critical care team on-call to consider interventions such as renal replacement therapy.

Lastly, the patient takes ramipril and spironolactone regularly, both of which can cause hyperkalaemia – these drugs should be withheld for now and should probably be discontinued in the future.

History

A 65-year-old man attended his GP surgery for a routine clinical review. He had been feeling well and had not experienced any recent illnesses. His past medical history included type 2 diabetes mellitus, which the patient had been attempting to control with dietary and other lifestyle modifications over the preceding 6 months, and hypertension. His regular medications were ramipril 5 mg OD and amlodipine 5 mg OD. He had no known drug allergies. He worked as a window cleaner, drank 20 units of alcohol weekly and was a current smoker of 10 cigarettes daily.

Examination

On examination, the patient appeared overweight but otherwise well. Systems examination was unremarkable.

Results

Bloods: WCC 5.7, Hb 139, Plt 341, Na 140, K 4.0, Creat 77 (eGFR 69), HbA1c 60 mmol/L

Question

Based on the above results, which of the following options is most appropriate?

Advise a further 6 months of lifestyle modifications (improving diet, increasing exercise)	☐
Commence gliclazide 40 mg OD and titrate the dose up over the coming weeks	☐
Commence metformin 500 mg OD and titrate the dose up over the coming weeks	☐
Commence pioglitazone 15 mg OD and titrate the dose up over the coming weeks	☐
Commence a multiple daily injection basal-bolus insulin regimen	☐

ANSWER

Advise a further 6 months of lifestyle modifications (improving diet, increasing exercise)	☐
Commence gliclazide 40 mg OD and titrate the dose up over the coming weeks	☐
Commence metformin 500 mg OD and titrate the dose up over the coming weeks	X
Commence pioglitazone 15 mg OD and titrate the dose up over the coming weeks	☐
Commence a multiple daily injection basal-bolus insulin regimen	☐

Metformin is currently recommended as the first choice for initial treatment for all patients with type 2 diabetes mellitus. Metformin is a biguanide medication that acts to reduce glucose synthesis within the liver. It additionally improves the body's sensitivity to endogenous insulin and reduces gastrointestinal absorption of glucose.

Following initiation of metformin treatment, the patient should be encouraged to monitor the blood glucose readings and the metformin can be uptitrated as needed. The HbA1c should be repeated in approximately 3-months' time, and further medication, such as a sulphonylurea (e.g. gliclazide) can be added in at this point. If glucose control remains poor, a further oral agent, or an insulin regimen may be commenced. The HbA1c (glycated haemoglobin) concentration represents general glucose control over the period of weeks to months and can be used to guide changes to diabetic therapies.

Lifestyle improvements, such as smoking cessation, healthy eating and regular exercise should be encouraged and a dietician referral or a 'keep fit' support group may help. Improvements in glycaemic control will reduce the risk of developing microvascular complications, including retinopathy, neuropathy and nephropathy, and macrovascular complications, including ischaemic heart disease, stroke and peripheral vascular disease.

History

A 72-year-old woman was brought to hospital after slipping on a wet floor and hurting her right knee. She denied any chest pain, palpitations, headache, shortness of breath or generalised weakness prior to the fall. Her past medical history included atrial fibrillation and glaucoma. She had no known allergies and her regular medications were: 3 mg warfarin OD, bisoprolol 2.5 mg OD, and latanoprost eye drops – 2 drops in her right eye OD. She was a retired musician, lived alone and was fully independent. She did not drink alcohol and had never smoked.

Examination

On examination, the patient appeared well and was fully orientated to time, place and person. Her heart rate was 60 bpm and irregularly irregular, her blood pressure was 120/80 mmHg (there was no postural drop) and her heart sounds were dual with no audible murmurs. Her chest was clear. Her abdomen was soft and non-tender. There was a small haematoma overlying her right knee joint but movement was fully preserved.

Results

Bloods: WCC 8.5, Hb 119, Plt 158, Na 140, K 4.0, Creat 50, CRP 13, INR 8.2

Question

Which *one* of the following options is most appropriate in this case?

Withhold the next dose of warfarin and re-check the INR the following day	☐
Administer phytomenadione 2 mg IV and re-check the INR in 4–6 h	☐
Administer phytomenadione 5 mg IV and re-check the INR in 4–6 h	☐
Administer phytomenadione 5 mg PO and re-check the INR in 4–6 h	☐
Administer fresh frozen plasma 12 mg/kg and re-check the INR in 4–6 h	☐

ANSWER

Withhold the next dose of warfarin and re-check the INR the following day	☐
Administer phytomenadione 2 mg IV and re-check the INR in 4–6 h	X
Administer phytomenadione 5 mg IV and re-check the INR in 4–6 h	☐
Administer phytomenadione 5 mg PO and re-check the INR in 4–6 h	☐
Administer fresh frozen plasma 12 mg/kg and re-check the INR in 4–6 h	☐

Warfarin is a vitamin K antagonist that inhibits the production of vitamin K-dependent clotting factors.

The patient has signs of minor bleeding (a right knee haematoma) and an INR >8.0 – the most appropriate treatment in this case, as per British National Formulary, is to administer phytomenadione (vitamin K) 2 mg intravenously. The INR should be rechecked 4–6 h later. Local guidelines may vary, so if you are unsure then the on-call haematology team should be contacted.

If the patient had signs of major bleeding, then both intravenous phytomenadione and fresh frozen plasma or dried prothrombin complex would be the appropriate therapy. If the patient had an INR <8.0 or no signs of bleeding then it would be appropriate to withhold the next 2–3 days' doses of warfarin and monitor the INR without giving phytomenadione.

History

A 30-year-old man was brought to hospital with generalised tonic clonic seizures. The seizure had commenced 5 min earlier and he had already received treatment with intravenous lorazepam (4 mg) and was given 5 mg diazepam intravenously upon arrival to the emergency department. There was evidence of tongue biting and he had been incontinent of urine. The patient was accompanied by his partner who reported that he had a known history of epilepsy, for which he usually took levetiracetam 500 mg BD. He worked as a civil servant and lived with his partner. He did not smoke cigarettes, drank approximately 5–6 units of alcohol per week and did not use recreational drugs.

Examination

On examination, the patient was unresponsive. There were jerking movements of the upper and lower limbs, consistent with a generalised tonic clonic seizure.

Question

After 25 min, the patient's seizure continued. Prescribe an appropriate medication to treat this ongoing seizure. The patient is estimated to weigh 80 kg.

ONCE ONLY MEDICATIONS									
Date	Medication	Dose	Route	Time of dose	Signature	Prescriber	Given by	Time given	Pharmacy

ANSWER

ONCE ONLY MEDICATIONS									
Date	Medication	Dose	Route	Time of dose	Signature	Prescriber	Given by	Time given	Pharmacy
01/01/20	PHENYTOIN	1.6 g	IV	12:00	*A Doctor*	A DOCTOR			

After 25 min of seizure activity (either continuous or recurring), and failure to respond to benzodiazepines, the patient is considered to be in status epilepticus. This should be treated with intravenous phenytoin sodium, fosphenytoin sodium, or phenobarbital sodium. In most hospitals, phenytoin is the agent of choice to treat status epilepticus.

In status epilepticus, phenytoin is prescribed at an initial dose of 20 mg/kg (up to a maximum of 2 g).

Question

Of these commonly prescribed medications, identify the *two* that have dosage errors:

Aspirin	75 mg	PO	OD	☐
Dalteparin	5000 units	PO	OD	☐
Ibuprofen	400 mg	PO	TDS	☐
Omeprazole	40 mg	PO	OD	☐
Paracetamol	2 g	PO	QDS	☐
Sertraline	50 mg	PO	OD	☐
Zopiclone	3.75 mg	PO	ON	☐

ANSWER

Aspirin	75 mg	PO	OD	☐
Dalteparin	5000 units	PO	OD	X
Ibuprofen	400 mg	PO	TDS	☐
Omeprazole	40 mg	PO	OD	☐
Paracetamol	2 g	PO	QDS	X
Sertraline	50 mg	PO	OD	☐
Zopiclone	3.75 mg	PO	ON	☐

Enoxaparin is a low molecular weight heparin and should be administered subcutaneously, not orally.

Paracetamol should be prescribed at a maximum of 1 g QDS – anything above this is considered to be an overdose.

History

A 68-year-old woman presented to her general practitioner complaining of a 2-week history of ankle swelling. Her past medical history included hypertension, iron deficiency anaemia, anxiety and restless legs syndrome. Her regular medications are listed below. She was a retired estate agent and lived with her partner. She drank approximately 14 units of alcohol per week and had never smoked.

Examination

The patient appeared well. Her heart rate was 60 bpm and her blood pressure was 128/84 mmHg. Her chest was clear and her abdomen was soft and non-tender. There was mild pitting oedema around the ankles but no peripheral oedema elsewhere.

Results

Bloods: WCC 7.3, Hb 130, Plt 188, Na 138, K 4.0, Creat 60, CRP <1, NT pro-BNP 120 (reference range <300 ng/L)

ECG: normal sinus rhythm, no evidence of left ventricular hypertrophy

Question

The general practitioner suspects that the peripheral oedema is an adverse effect related to her current medication. Which *two* of the medications below commonly cause peripheral oedema?

Amitriptyline	25 mg	PO	ON	☐
Amlodipine	10 mg	PO	OD	☐
Bendroflumethiazide	2.5 mg	PO	OD	☐
Bisoprolol	2.5 mg	PO	OD	☐
Ferrous sulfate	200 mg	PO	OD	☐
Pramipexole	500 µg	PO	OD	☐
Zopiclone	7.5 mg	PO	OD	☐

ANSWER

Amitriptyline	25 mg	PO	ON	☐
Amlodipine	10 mg	PO	OD	X
Bendroflumethiazide	2.5 mg	PO	OD	☐
Bisoprolol	2.5 mg	PO	OD	☐
Ferrous sulfate	200 mg	PO	OD	☐
Pramipexole	500 μg	PO	OD	X
Zopiclone	7.5 mg	PO	OD	☐

Calcium channel blockers, particularly the vasodilating dihydropyridines, such as amlodipine, are well recognised as a common cause of peripheral oedema. This potentially occurs due to calcium channel blockers modifying capillary permeability and thus redistributing fluid from the capillaries to the interstitial space.

There is additionally a strong association between the use of pramipexole, a non-ergot agonist at the dopamine D_2 and D_3 receptors, and the development of peripheral oedema.

Other drugs that are recognised to cause peripheral oedema include non-steroidal anti-inflammatory drugs (NSAIDs), pioglitazone, gabapentin and pregabalin.

History

A 67-year-old woman presented to the emergency department complaining of difficulty in breathing. She had experienced increasing shortness of breath over the preceding weeks and this was exacerbated by lying down in bed at night. She also complained of worsening leg swelling over the previous fortnight. Her past medical history included hypertension and osteoarthritis. Her regular medications are listed below. She lived with her partner, smoked 10 cigarettes daily and drank approximately 20 units of alcohol per week.

Examination

The patient appeared visibly dyspnoeic. She was afebrile. Her heart rate was 94 bpm and her blood pressure was 148/90 mmHg. Her heart sounds were normal. There were crackles up to the mid zones of her chest bilaterally. Her respiratory rate was 20 and her peripheral oxygen saturations (SpO$_2$) were 93% on room air. There was bilateral pitting oedema up to the level of her thighs.

Results

Bloods: WCC 8.4, Hb 139, Plt 275, Na 140, K 4.1, Creat 71, NT-proBNP 4760 (reference range <300 ng/L)

Chest X-ray

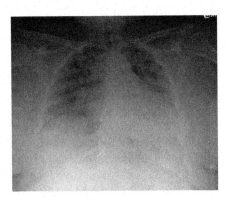

Questions

In view of the above information:

1. Which *two* of the patient's regular medications should be stopped?
2. Which *one* of the patient's regular medications should be uptitrated, as tolerated?

				1	2
Atorvastatin	80 mg	PO	ON	☐	☐
Bisoprolol	10 mg	PO	OD	☐	☐
Dihydrocodeine	30 mg	PO	QDS	☐	☐
Ibuprofen	200 mg	PO	TDS	☐	☐
Paracetamol	1 g	PO	QDS	☐	☐
Ramipril	5 mg	PO	OD	☐	☐
Verapamil	120 mg	PO	OD	☐	☐

ANSWERS

				1	2
Atorvastatin	80 mg	PO	ON	☐	☐
Bisoprolol	10 mg	PO	OD	☐	☐
Dihydrocodeine	30 mg	PO	QDS	☐	☐
Ibuprofen	200 mg	PO	TDS	X	☐
Paracetamol	1 g	PO	QDS	☐	☐
Ramipril	5 mg	PO	OD	☐	X
Verapamil	120 mg	PO	OD	X	☐

The patient has described shortness of breath, orthopnoea and ankle swelling and systems examination identified signs of peripheral and pulmonary oedema. Her blood results show an elevated BNP level and her chest X-ray shows patchy opacification bilaterally, in keeping with pulmonary oedema. These symptoms, signs and investigations are consistent with a diagnosis of pulmonary oedema.

Renal prostaglandins facilitate urinary sodium excretion and thus increase water excretion. Non-steroidal anti-inflammatory drugs (NSAIDs) inhibit the synthesis of prostaglandins and can worsen fluid retention in patients with heart failure. NSAIDs, particularly COX-2 inhibitors, are also associated with an increased risk of cardiovascular events.

Calcium channel blockers have negative inotropic effects. The non-dihydropyridines, in particular, reduce cardiac output and slow the heart rate; they should be avoided in patients with heart failure as they can exacerbate the condition.

Beta blockers were previously thought to be contraindicated in heart failure, but newer evidence shows that they are actually beneficial in the management of chronic heart failure. Their role in acute heart failure is less clear, but current guidance suggests that patients who are already established on beta blockers should continue on these during acute heart failure. Patients with chronic heart failure should be prescribed the maximum dose of beta blocker (usually bisoprolol) and ACE inhibitor (usually ramipril) that can be tolerated, as both drug classes have been shown to reduce left ventricular remodelling in these patients, and some beta blockers may even reverse cardiac remodelling.

History

An 86-year-old woman was reviewed by her general practitioner following some recent changes to her medications. She felt well and had not experienced any chest pain, shortness of breath or falls/collapses over recent weeks. Her past medical history included atrial fibrillation, hypertension, ischaemic heart disease and heart failure. Her regular medications were: ramipril 5 mg OD, bisoprolol 5 mg OD, isosorbide mononitrate (modified release) 30 mg OD, and she had recently commenced digoxin, which had been uptitrated to 250 μg OD. She lived with her husband, smoked 10 cigarettes daily and drank approximately 18 units of alcohol per week.

Examination

The patient appeared generally well. Her heart rate was 66 bpm and her blood pressure was 134/70 mmHg. Her chest was clear and she had mild ankle oedema.

Results

Bloods: Na 137, K 4.1, Creat 45, digoxin level 2.3 μg/L (reference interval 0.8 to 2.2 μg/L)

ECG: atrial fibrillation at a rate of approximately 60 beats/min

Question

Based on the above information, which *one* of the following options would you recommend to her general practitioner?

Administer digoxin-specific antibody immediately	☐
Cease digoxin therapy and advise the patient she is unable to continue taking the medication	☐
Continue prescribing the current dose of digoxin (250 μg OD)	☐
Withhold the next 1–2 doses of digoxin and then reduce the dose to 125 μg OD	☐

ANSWER

Administer digoxin-specific antibody immediately	☐
Cease digoxin therapy and advise the patient she is unable to continue taking the medication	☐
Continue prescribing the current dose of digoxin (250 µg OD)	☐
Withhold the next 1–2 doses of digoxin and then reduce the dose to 125 µg OD	X

The digoxin level is mildly elevated, but it is important to remember that digoxin has a narrow therapeutic index so toxicity can develop at levels that are only slightly above the reference interval. The correct option would be to withhold the next 1–2 doses of digoxin and then reduce the dose down to 125 µg daily. A repeat digoxin level should be sent 1–2 weeks later.

The patient has no symptoms or signs of digoxin toxicity (bradycardia, heart block, or other arrhythmias, nausea and anorexia, collapse, yellow tint to vision or hyperkalaemia) and treatment with digoxin-specific antibody is therefore not required.

History

A 17-year-old man was brought to hospital with abdominal pain and vomiting of 12 h duration. He had a past medical history of type 1 diabetes mellitus. He reported that he had missed several doses of his regular insulin whilst on a school trip.

Examination

The patient was awake and alert. His heart rate was 90 bpm and his blood pressure was 120/80 mmHg. His abdomen was soft but mildly tender throughout.

Results

A venous blood gas showed: pH 7.14, HCO_3 14, lactate 6.2, glucose 'high'

Blood ketones: 4.3 mmol/L

Bloods: WCC 10.4, Hb 168, Plt 430, Na 140, K 5.6, urea 15.6, Creat 88, glucose 28

Questions

1. Which two treatments below should be administered immediately?
2. Assuming he recovers well, which one treatment option will the patient likely commence after 12–24 h?

	1	2
Sodium chloride 0.9% 1000 mLs IV over 60 min	☐	☐
Sodium chloride 0.9% 1000 mLs IV over 15 min	☐	☐
Glucose 5% 1000 mLs IV over 60 min	☐	☐
Glucose 5% 1000 mLs IV over 15 min	☐	☐
Fixed rate insulin intravenous infusion 0.1 unit/kg/h	☐	☐
Fixed rate insulin subcutaneous infusion 0.1 unit/kg/h	☐	☐
Variable rate intravenous insulin infusion	☐	☐
The patient's regular insulin dose	☐	☐

ANSWERS

	1	2
Sodium chloride 0.9% 1000 mLs IV over 60 minutes	X	☐
Sodium chloride 0.9% 1000 mLs IV over 15 min	☐	☐
Glucose 5% 1000 mLs IV over 60 min	☐	☐
Glucose 5% 1000 mLs IV over 15 min	☐	☐
Fixed rate insulin intravenous infusion 0.1unit/kg/h	X	☐
Fixed rate insulin subcutaneous infusion 0.1unit/kg/h	☐	☐
Variable rate intravenous insulin infusion ('sliding scale')	☐	☐
The patient's regular insulin dose	☐	X

Firstly, it is important to consider that many hospitals have local protocols in place to guide the management of diabetic ketoacidosis (DKA) and hyperglycemic hyperosmolar state (HHS) and these should be adhered to where appropriate, with further advice obtained from a specialist diabetes or endocrine team as needed.

In this case, the patient's blood results meet the criteria for a diagnosis of DKA: (1) pH <7.3 and/ or HCO_3 < 15 mmol/L, (2) blood glucose >11 mmol/L, and (3) blood ketones > 3 mmol/L and/or urine ketones ++ or greater.

In patients who have no significant comorbidities, are hemodynamically stable, have a venous pH >7.10, and a potassium level >3.5 mmol/L, 1000 mL 0.9% sodium chloride should be administered over 60 min. Potassium supplementation may be required. A fixed rate intravenous insulin infusion at a rate of 0.1 units/kg/h should be also commenced at this point.

The patient's glucose levels, venous pH, ketone levels and potassium levels will guide further management over the next 12 h.

Following recovery from DKA, the patient can usually take their regular insulin dose and the intravenous insulin infusion can be discontinued 30 min later – if a diabetes or endocrine specialist team is available, their advice should be sought to guide re-initiation of regular subcutaneous insulin therapy.

History
A 42-year-old woman attended her antenatal clinic for a routine check-up. She was 6-months pregnant and thus far had not experienced any complications associated with this pregnancy. This was her first pregnancy. She had no known past medical history and took no regular medications aside from vitamin supplements. She worked as a pharmacist and did not drink alcohol or smoke.

Examination
The patient appeared generally well. Her blood pressure was measured three times and was noted to be: 159/95 mmHg, 156/90 mmHg and 152/88 mmHg. There was no significant difference between the blood pressure readings using the left and right arms. There was no peripheral oedema. Systems examination was otherwise unremarkable and the pregnancy was deemed to be progressing appropriately.

Results
Urine dip: no leucocytes, no erythrocytes, no protein, no nitrites

Bloods: WCC 5.1, Hb 109, Plt 391, Na 137, K 3.8, Creat 47

Question
The obstetrician advised that the patient should commence an antihypertensive agent. Which *two* medications would be appropriate to prescribe?

Candesartan	☐
Labetalol	☐
Methyldopa	☐
Perindopril	☐
Ramipril	☐

ANSWER

Candesartan	☐
Labetalol	X
Methyldopa	X
Perindopril	☐
Ramipril	☐

It is important to exclude pre-eclampsia in pregnant patients with hypertension, particularly in the second half of pregnancy. Based on the urine dip test, this patient does not have any protein in her urine, which makes pre-eclampsia less likely. The patient should still be advised to seek medical support if she develops a headache, peripheral oedema or visual changes.

Oral labetalol is usually given as the first-line agent in treating moderate hypertension (150/100–159/109 mmHg). Methyldopa and nifedipine are typical second-line antihypertensives.

ACE inhibitors and angiotensin II receptor blockers are associated with an increased risk of congenital abnormalities and should be stopped as soon as a pregnancy is confirmed. Ideally, women of child-bearing potential should not be prescribed these medications unless suitable alternatives are not available.

Beta-blockers, calcium channel antagonists (aside from nifedipine) and diuretics should be avoided ideally but are not contraindicated in pregnancy.

History

An 82-year-old man was admitted to hospital with symptoms of cough and fever. He was diagnosed with an aspiration pneumonia secondary to impaired swallowing function. He was due to have a nasogastric tube sited the following day but will need intravenous fluid hydration overnight.

Question

You need to prescribe a 1 L bag of 0.9% sodium chloride to run over 8 h. The fluid will be administered via a controlled-rate infusion pump.

At what rate should the infusion be administered?

The infusion should be administered at a rate of ☐ mL/min.

ANSWER

You will administer 1000 mL of fluid over 8 h. This is equivalent to 125 mL/h, or 2.08 mL/min.

The answer is 2 mL/min.

History
A 6-year-old boy was brought to his general practitioner by his parents after developing a fever and a sore throat. He had been feeling unwell for 2 days. His younger sister had experienced similar symptoms earlier. The patient had no past medical history, had no known drug allergies and did not take any regular medications. He lived with his parents and two siblings and attended the local school.

Examination
On examination, the patient appeared clinically well. His temperature was 37.8°C. His throat appeared erythematous but the tonsils were not enlarged. Systems examination was otherwise unremarkable.

Question
The patient's parents asked whether there were any 'over-the-counter' medicines that they could purchase to relieve his symptoms of sore throat and fever. Which *one* of the medications below should the parents be advised to avoid, where possible, in children under the age of 12 years?

Aspirin dispersible tablet	☐
Benzydamine throat spray	☐
Benzocaine throat spray	☐
Ibuprofen tablet	☐
Paracetamol dispersible tablet	☐

ANSWER

Aspirin dispersible tablet	X
Benzydamine throat spray	☐
Benzocaine throat spray	☐
Ibuprofen tablet	☐
Paracetamol dispersible tablet	☐

There is a strong association between the use of aspirin in children with viral illnesses and the development of the rare condition, Reye's syndrome. Reye's syndrome is characterised by encephalopathy and liver failure secondary to mitochondrial dysfunction.

Paracetamol and ibuprofen should instead be used as antipyretics/analgesics in children under the age of 12 years. Anaesthetic (benzocaine) and NSAID (benzydamine) throat sprays and anaesthetic lozenges may also provide relief.

History

A 45-year-old man attended a routine assessment at the sexual health clinic, where a sexually transmitted infection screen identified that the patient's blood was positive for HIV. He was referred to the local HIV clinic and commenced anti-retroviral therapy later that week. The patient denied experiencing any symptoms and reported that he had been well over recent months. He had no significant past medical history and took no regular medications. He worked as a librarian and lived with his partner. He drank 10 units of alcohol per week and had never smoked.

Examination

The patient appeared clinically well. Systems examination was unremarkable. Of note, there was no palpable cervical, axillary or inguinal lymphadenopathy, and there was no oral candidiasis.

Results

Bloods: WCC 3.9 (neutrophils 3.2, lymphocytes 0.5), Hb 145, Plt 205, Na 137, K 3.8, Creat 72, Bili 16, ALT 24, ALP 45

HIV viral load: 84,000

CD4 count: 82 (reference range 500–1400 cells/mm^3)

Question

Based on the patient's blood results, you are asked to prescribe pneumocystis pneumonia prophylaxis using the chart below:

			Date					
DRUG (print approved name)		Dose	6					
			8					
Signature	Date	Route	12					
Print name	Bleep	Pharmacy	14					
			18					
Additional information			22					

ANSWER

DRUG (print approved name)		Dose	Date						
CO-TRIMOXAZOLE		480 mg	6						
			(8)						
Signature	Date	Route	12						
A Doctor	01/01/20	PO							
Print name	Bleep	Pharmacy	14						
A DOCTOR	1234								
			18						
Additional information									
PCP prophylaxis			22						

The patient has a CD4 count <200 and a high HIV viral load and is therefore at risk of developing opportunistic infections, including pneumocystis pneumonia (commonly referred to as 'PCP'), which is an infection with the fungus *Pneumocystis jirovecii*.

PCP prophylaxis should be commenced until the patient's immune function has recovered. The first-line treatment option is co-trimoxazole, a combination drug consisting of trimethoprim and sulphamethoxazole. The British National Formulary lists the standard dose as 960 mg (160 mg trimethoprim/800 mg sulphamethoxazole), to be reduced to 480 mg if this dose is not tolerated, but most HIV centres advise that patients take 480 mg OD, as this dose has a similar efficacy with fewer side effects. Both 480 mg OD and 960 mg OD would therefore be correct answers.

Second-line PCP prophylaxis in patients who are unable to tolerate co-trimoxazole is usually dapsone 100 mg OD or atovaquone 750 mg BD.

History

A 72-year-old woman was reviewed by her general practitioner after reporting increasing symptoms of shortness of breath and cough over recent weeks following several changes to her regular medications. Her general practitioner suspected that she was experiencing an exacerbation of her asthma and commenced a 5-day course of prednisolone 40 mg PO OD. Upon review, the patient stated that she had not noticed any improvement in her symptoms of shortness of breath but now also felt increasingly distressed and agitated. Her past medical history was significant for anxiety, hay fever and asthma. Her regular medications at the time of her review are listed below.

Examination

The patient appeared generally well. There was a mild, polyphonic expiratory wheeze heard throughout her chest.

Questions

1. Select the *one* medication that is most likely to have caused the patient's shortness of breath and wheeze to have developed.
2. Select the *one* medication that is most likely exacerbated the patient's anxiety symptoms.

				1	2
Carbocisteine	375 mg	PO	OD	☐	☐
Diazepam	5 mg	PO	OD	☐	☐
Escitalopram	10 mg	PO	OD	☐	☐
Prednisolone	40 mg	PO	OD	☐	☐
Prochlorperazine	10 mg	PO	BD	☐	☐
Propranolol	40 mg	PO	OD	☐	☐
Zopiclone	7.5 mg	PO	ON	☐	☐

ANSWERS

				1	2
Carbocisteine	375 mg	PO	OD	☐	☐
Diazepam	5 mg	PO	OD	☐	☐
Escitalopram	10 mg	PO	OD	☐	☐
Prednisolone	40 mg	PO	OD	☐	X
Prochlorperazine	10 mg	PO	BD	☐	☐
Propranolol	40 mg	PO	OD	X	☐
Zopiclone	7.5 mg	PO	ON	☐	☐

1. Beta blockers can be classified as either: (i) cardioselective, primarily inhibiting β receptors within the heart or (ii) non-cardioselective, inhibiting all β receptors. Propranolol is a non-selective beta blocker and will thus inhibit β_2-adrenoceptors that promote bronchodilation, potentially leading to bronchoconstriction.

   Cardioselective beta blockers, such as bisoprolol, are generally safe to prescribe in mild, well-controlled asthma if there is no suitable alternative agent. Non-cardioselective beta blockers, such as propranolol, should be avoided in asthmatic patients, or those with chronic obstructive pulmonary disease wherever possible.

2. The patient has recently commenced a course of prednisolone. Corticosteroids commonly cause changes in mood, including anxiety and agitation, and can precipitate psychotic episodes in some patients.

History

A 74-year-old woman presented to the emergency department with shortness of breath and a cough. She described a 72-h history of feeling feverish with a dry cough and worsening shortness of breath. Her past medical history included type 2 diabetes mellitus and depression. She had no known drug allergies and her regular medications were metformin 500 mg OD and sertraline 50 mg OD. The patient lived alone and volunteered at a local animal shelter.

Examination

The patient appeared dyspnoeic and generally unwell. She was febrile (temperature 38.4°C) and tachycardic (HR 120 bpm). Her blood pressure was 110/75 mmHg. Her heart sounds were dual with no murmurs. On auscultation of the chest, there were crackles throughout the left mid and lower zones. Her abdomen was soft and non-tender.

Results

Rapid influenza diagnostic swab: positive for influenza A

Question

Based on the above results, please prescribe an appropriate therapy to reduce replication of influenza A.

DRUG (print approved name)		Dose	Date					
			6					
			8					
Signature	Date	Route	12					
Print name	Bleep	Pharmacy	14					
			18					
Additional information			22					

ANSWER

DRUG (print approved name)		Dose	Date						
OSELTAMIVIR		75 mg	6						
			(8)						
Signature	Date	Route	12						
A Doctor	01/01/20	PO							
Print name	Bleep	Pharmacy	14						
A DOCTOR	1234		(18)						
Additional information									
Confirmed influenza A, 10 day course			22						

Oseltamivir works by inhibiting viral neuraminidase and thus reducing the replication of influenza viruses. Oseltamivir is prescribed as a twice daily 75 mg oral dose in patients who have a confirmed influenza infection.

Oseltamivir is prescribed prophylactically as a once daily 75 mg oral dose in patients who have been exposed to other people with confirmed influenza and are either at increased risk of developing severe illness or are hospital inpatients (and thus could infect other patients).

History

A 27-year-old man was brought to hospital with a painful left leg. He had noticed increasing pain and swelling over his left thigh for several days. He had been feeling feverish and became lightheaded when he attempted to stand up. He had no significant past medical history and took no regular medications. The patient was a current intravenous drug user and injected heroin several times daily, with his left groin being his favoured injection site. He did not drink alcohol and did not use other recreational drugs. He had no fixed abode and usually sleeps in a hostel.

Examination

On examination, the patient was febrile (temperature 39.0°C) and appeared generally unwell. His heart sounds were dual with no murmurs, his heart rate was 100 bpm and his blood pressure was 100/70 mmHg. The left thigh appeared erythematous and swollen and the skin was hot to touch. There was a yellow-green exudate oozing from a sinus tract in his left groin.

Results

Bloods: WCC 18.7, Hb 139, Plt 298, Na 142, K 4.2, Creat 72 (eGFR 90), CRP 281

Ultrasound Doppler of left leg: no evidence of a deep vein thrombosis

Swab from left groin: Gram positive cocci – resistant to penicillins, sensitive to vancomycin

Blood cultures: no bacterial growth

Question

The patient was initially prescribed intravenous flucloxacillin, however, once the microbiology results were available, intravenous vancomycin was prescribed instead. Which of the following options is the most appropriate way to monitor the serum concentrations of vancomycin?

A vancomycin level should be taken after the first dose	☐
A vancomycin level should be taken immediately after the third dose	☐
A vancomycin level should be taken immediately before the fourth dose	☐
Vancomycin levels are not required as this patient has normal renal function	☐

ANSWER

A vancomycin level should be taken after the first dose	☐
A vancomycin level should be taken immediately after the third dose	☐
A vancomycin level should be taken immediately before the fourth dose	X
Vancomycin levels are not required as this patient has normal renal function	☐

Vancomycin has a narrow therapeutic index, with reduced efficacy and increased rates of bacterial resistance developing at vancomycin levels below the reference interval and an increased risk of toxicity (nephrotoxicity and ototoxicity) at levels above the reference interval.

In patients with normal renal function, vancomycin can be dosed twice daily. Vancomycin trough doses are initially taken once steady state is achieved – this is usually after the third dose. Vancomycin trough levels are used in the majority of cases, and the serum sample should be obtained up to 30 min before the next dose – that is, the first vancomycin level is taken ≤30 min before the fourth dose. The next dose should then be given as the serum level will not be back in time to guide the fourth dose. In some cases, for example, bacteraemia, the microbiology and pharmacy teams may additionally request peak levels which are taken 1–2 h post-dose.

The vancomycin dose will be withheld, continued or up/downtitrated, based on the vancomycin trough level. A typical target vancomycin trough level is 15–20 mg/L. In patients with normal renal function and an initial vancomycin trough level within the reference range, monitoring can be performed less frequently.

History

A 60-year-old man attended his general practitioner to discuss results of recent blood tests. He had initially attended for a routine review 6 months earlier after reaching 60 years of age, and was noted to have an elevated body mass index at that point. He had since attempted to improve his diet by eating more fruit and vegetables and had also joined a gym. He reported feeling generally well and had not experienced any illnesses over the past few months. He had no past medical history aside from a previous knee injury and he took no regular medications. He worked as a stone sawyer, drank 4–6 units of alcohol per week and had recently stopped smoking.

Results

Bloods: WCC 7.1, Hb 159, Plt 275, Na 140, K 3.9, Creat 70, Bili 12, ALT 19, ALP 40, LDL 5.0 (<3 mmol/L), HDL 1.0 (>1.2 mmol/L)

Case progression

The patient's general practitioner discussed the above results with the patient and he felt that he would be unable to make further lifestyle modifications. They decided that the patient should commence lipid-modifying therapy.

Question

Prescribe an appropriate lipid-modifying drug below.

DRUG (print approved name)		Dose	Date						
			6						
			8						
Signature	Date	Route	12						
Print name	Bleep	Pharmacy	14						
			18						
Additional information			22						

ANSWER

DRUG (print approved name)		Dose	Date						
ATORVASTATIN		20 mg	6						
			8						
Signature	Date	Route	12						
A Doctor	01/01/20	PO							
Print name	Bleep	Pharmacy	14						
A DOCTOR	1234		18						
Additional information			(22)						

The patient's blood results show that he has elevated serum LDL levels and is thus at increased risk of developing cardiovascular disease. A cardiovascular risk calculator, such as the QRISK®3-2018 calculator, can be used to help guide physicians as to whether lipid-modifying therapy should be commenced. As with all medications, lipid-modifying therapies are associated with several adverse effects and should thus only be prescribed for patients who are likely to derive considerable benefit from these therapies.

The National Institute for Health and Care Excellence (NICE) recommends commencing one of the following high-intensity statins as the first-line agent for primary prevention of cardiovascular disease:

1. Atorvastatin 20–80 mg ON
2. Rosuvastatin 10–40 mg ON
3. Simvastatin 80 mg ON

All of the above options would be appropriate answers. The example of atorvastatin 20 mg ON is shown above.

History

A 75-year-old man was admitted to hospital with community-acquired pneumonia. Whilst he was in hospital, he was transferred to an elderly care ward, where his regular medications were reviewed – several drugs were stopped but he also commenced new drugs. Six days into his hospital admission, the patient developed jaundice and abdominal pain. His blood showed abnormal liver function (see below). An abdominal ultrasound scan was unremarkable and you are asked to review his medications to establish whether he could have a drug-induced liver injury.

Results

Bloods: Bili 49, ALT 60, ALP 210, Albumin 30, GGT 196, INR 1.2

Question

Which *two* of the drugs below are most likely responsible for the patient's potential hepatotoxicity?

Alendronic acid	☐
Amoxicillin-clavulanate	☐
Aspirin	☐
Carbocisteine	☐
Digoxin	☐
Prednisolone	☐
Simvastatin	☐

ANSWER

Alendronic acid	☐
Amoxicillin-clavulanate	X
Aspirin	☐
Carbocisteine	☐
Digoxin	☐
Prednisolone	☐
Simvastatin	X

Drug-induced acute liver injuries are triggered by many medications, although amoxicillin-clavulanate (also known as co-amoxiclav) is thought to be the most common cause in Europe and the United States. Patients with amoxicillin-clavulanate hepatotoxicity typically present with a cholestatic picture, as in this case. Patients taking the combination of amoxicillin-clavulanate are around six times more likely to develop hepatotoxicity compared to those taking amoxicillin only. Although cholestatic jaundice is the usual presentation of amoxicillin-clavulanate hepatotoxicity, patients may also develop raised aminotransferase concentrations, indicating hepatocellular injury.

Simvastatin, as with other statins, frequently induces a mild, transient rise in serum aminotransferase concentrations in up to 5% of patients. Approximately 1% of patients will develop a significant liver injury, although the mechanism of this is not fully understood.

Other common causes of drug-induced liver injury include (but are not limited to): amiodarone, ciprofloxacin, fluconazole, isoniazid, methyldopa, oral contraceptives, paracetamol, rifampicin and sodium valproate.

Patients should also be questioned regarding their use of over-the-counter medicines, recreational drugs and herbal medicines, many of which can cause acute kidney or liver injuries.

History

A 66-year-old woman was admitted to hospital with fever, dysuria and right flank pain. Her urine dip was positive for nitrites and she was diagnosed with pyelonephritis.

Question

You are asked to prescribe intravenous gentamicin at a dose of 5 mg/kg to treat the patient's pyelonephritis. Gentamicin ampoules contain 80 mg/mL and should be mixed with 0.9% sodium chloride to make a solution of 1 mg/mL gentamicin.

The patient weighs 60 kg and has normal renal function.

The infusion should be administered over 60 min. At what rate should the controlled-rate infusion pump run?

The gentamicin infusion should run at ☐ mL/min.

ANSWER

The patient weighs 60 kg and will therefore need 300 mg gentamicin over 60 min.

Gentamicin vials contain 80 mg/2 mL but are diluted with 0.9% sodium chloride to prepare a solution that is at a concentration of 1 mg/mL. A 300 mL solution should therefore be prepared and administered over 60 min.

The answer is 5 mL/min.

CASE 70: PROVIDING INFORMATION 3

History

A 55-year-old man was admitted to hospital with shortness of breath and a cough productive of green sputum. His past medical history included type 2 diabetes and chronic obstructive pulmonary disease. His regular medications were metformin 500 mg BD, a beclometasone/formoterol 200/6 inhaler 2 puffs BD and a salbutamol 200 µg inhaler 2 puffs BD. He worked as a security officer, was an ex-smoker with a 10-pack year history and drank approximately 6 units of alcohol per week.

Question

The patient was diagnosed with an exacerbation of chronic obstructive pulmonary disease and was advised to commence a course of prednisolone 30 mg PO OD. Select the *two* most appropriate statements below that should be explained to the patient.

Prednisolone may cause a rise in his blood glucose levels	☐
Prednisolone may cause a fall in his blood glucose levels	☐
Prednisolone is contraindicated in patients with type 2 diabetes mellitus	☐
Prednisolone should be avoided in patients who receive inhaled steroids	☐
The patient may need an alternative dose of metformin whilst he is taking prednisolone	☐

ANSWER

Prednisolone may cause a rise in his blood glucose levels	X
Prednisolone may cause a fall in his blood glucose levels	☐
Prednisolone is contraindicated in patients with type 2 diabetes mellitus	☐
Prednisolone should be avoided in patients who receive inhaled steroids	☐
The patient may need an alternative dose of metformin whilst he is taking prednisolone	X

Corticosteroids, such as prednisolone, promote hepatic gluconeogenesis and increase insulin resistance via a variety of mechanisms, including increasing visceral adipose tissue deposition and enhancing the mobilisation of free fatty acids into the circulation.

Patients who have underlying diabetes mellitus (type 1 or type 2) typically experience a rise in their blood glucose levels once starting corticosteroid therapy and their diabetic medications may need to be uptitrated as a consequence.

Patients who have impaired glycaemic control may develop steroid-induced diabetes whilst taking corticosteroids – this often resolves following cessation of the corticosteroid therapy, but such patients have an increased risk of developing type 2 diabetes mellitus in later life.

Question

Of these commonly prescribed antibiotics, identify the *two* that have dosage errors:

Amoxicillin	625 mg	PO	TDS	☐
Clarithromycin	500 mg	PO	BD	☐
Doxycycline	200 mg	PO	OD	☐
Gentamicin	300 mg	PO	OD	☐
Levofloxacin	500 mg	PO	BD	☐
Penicillin V	250 mg	PO	BD	☐
Trimethoprim	200 mg	PO	BD	☐

ANSWER

Amoxicillin	625 mg	PO	TDS	X
Clarithromycin	500 mg	PO	BD	☐
Doxycycline	200 mg	PO	OD	☐
Gentamicin	300 mg	PO	OD	X
Levofloxacin	500 mg	PO	BD	☐
Penicillin V	250 mg	PO	BD	☐
Trimethoprim	200 mg	PO	BD	☐

Gentamicin is not available in an oral formulation and is typically prescribed as either an intravenous infusion/injection or an intramuscular injection, although the intrathecal and topical routes are appropriate in certain clinical situations.

Amoxicillin is prescribed as either 500 mg or 1000 mg oral tablets in adult patients. Amoxicillin-clavulanate (co-amoxiclav), however, is available as a 625 mg oral tablet.

CASE 72: DRUG MONITORING 4

History

A 68-year-old woman was admitted to hospital with fever and right flank pain of 48-h duration. She had also felt nauseated and experienced dysuria for the preceding 72 h. She had no past medical history and her only regular medication was hormone replacement therapy. She worked as a journalist, drank approximately 8 units of alcohol per week and had never smoked.

Examination

The patient was febrile (temperature 39.0°C). Her heart rate was 120 bpm and her blood pressure was 110/60 mmHg. Her abdomen was soft with mild left flank tenderness on deep palpation.

Results

Bloods: WCC 16.3, Hb 130, Plt 199, Na 140, K 4.4, Creat 55 (eGFR 121), CRP 300

Case progression

The patient was diagnosed with pyelonephritis and commenced treatment with intravenous amoxicillin-clavulanate (co-amoxiclav). She also received a 'one off' intravenous infusion of gentamicin, dosed at 7 mg/kg.

Question

Despite initially improving, the patient becomes febrile again on the second day of her admission and experiences rigors. You are asked to prescribe a further dose of gentamicin for the patient. Which *one* of the statements below is most appropriate in this situation?

The patient has received an appropriate dose of gentamicin and does not need a further dose	☐
The patient has normal renal function and should thus be given another dose now	☐
The patient should have a serum gentamicin trough level taken and the next dose should then be given immediately	☐
The patient should have a serum gentamicin trough level taken and the next dose should then be withheld until the results are available	☐

ANSWER

The patient has received an appropriate dose of gentamicin and does not need a further dose	☐
The patient has normal renal function and should thus be given another dose now	☐
The patient should have a serum gentamicin trough level taken and the next dose should then be given immediately	☐
The patient should have a serum gentamicin trough level taken and the next dose should then be withheld until the results are available	X

Gentamicin has a narrow therapeutic window and severe adverse effects can develop following an overdose. Many hospitals will have local policies relating to the monitoring of serum gentamicin concentrations.

Generally, when used once daily to treat sepsis, gentamicin trough (pre-dose) concentrations are used to guide decisions regarding re-dosing, with further doses of gentamicin being withheld until the serum concentration is ≤1 mg/L.

Some hospitals advise that if the initial gentamicin level is ≤1 mg/L in patients who are 65 years of age or younger with normal, stable renal function, they may continue on a once daily gentamicin regimen with a trough (pre-dose) level taken twice weekly.

History

A 48-year-old woman was reviewed by her general practitioner after developing symptoms of weight gain and fatigue. She had been feeling generally unwell for several weeks. Her past medical history included type 1 diabetes mellitus and hypothyroidism. Her regular medications were: insulin (via a continuous pump), ferrous sulfate 200 mg OD and levothyroxine 75 µg OD. She worked as a diving instructor, did not smoke and did not drink alcohol.

Results

Bloods: WCC 5.5, Hb 130, Plt 250, Na 136, K 3.6, Creat 50, TSH 6.8 mIU/L (reference interval 0.2–5.0 mIU/L)

Question

Based on the above information, which *one* of the following options would you recommend to her general practitioner?

Cease levothyroxine therapy	☐
Continue prescribing the current dose of levothyroxine (75 µg OD)	☐
Increase the levothyroxine dose to 100 µg OD	☐
Reduce the levothyroxine dose to 50 µg OD	☐

ANSWER

Cease levothyroxine therapy	☐
Continue prescribing the current dose of levothyroxine (75 µg OD)	☐
Increase the levothyroxine dose to 100 µg OD	X
Reduce the levothyroxine dose to 50 µg OD	☐

The patient has symptoms of hypothyroidism (fatigue and weight gain) and her blood results confirm that her current dose of levothyroxine is not sufficient to maintain a normal TSH level. The levothyroxine dose should be increased to 100 µg OD and a repeat TSH level should be checked in 2–3 weeks' time. Both the TSH level and the patient's symptoms should be used to guide the levothyroxine dose titration.

History

A 28-year-old woman was admitted to hospital after becoming light-headed and short of breath when walking to work. She reported experiencing several episodes of light-headedness over recent days. The patient's last menstrual period began 5 days earlier. Her past medical history included menorrhagia secondary to fibroids. Her only regular medication was the combined oral contraceptive pill.

Examination

The patient appeared pale but otherwise well. Her heart rate was 70 bpm and her blood pressure was 122/75 mmHg (there was no postural drop in blood pressure). A full systems examination, including a digital rectal examination, was unremarkable.

Results

Bloods: WCC 4.3, Hb 83, MCV 72, Plt 203, Na 138, Creat 62, iron level 3.0 (reference range 12–28 μmol/L), vitamin B_{12} 530 (reference range 180–1000 pg/mL), folate 7 (reference range >4 ng/mL)

Question

Based on the above information from the options below, select the *one* most appropriate treatment for this patient:

Cyanocobalamin	1 mg	IM	One dose	☐
Ferric carboxymaltose	1 g	IV	One dose	☐
Ferrous sulfate	200 mg	PO	TDS	☐
Folic acid	5 mg	PO	OD	☐
Packed red cells	1 unit	IV	One dose	☐

ANSWER

Cyanocobalamin	1 mg	IM	One dose	☐
Ferric carboxymaltose	1 g	IV	One dose	X
Ferrous sulfate	200 mg	PO	TDS	☐
Folic acid	5 mg	PO	OD	☐
Packed red cells	1 unit	IV	One dose	☐

The patient has a significant iron deficiency anaemia that is likely to be secondary to menorrhagia. The patient is haemodynamically stable, appears well and has a haemoglobin level of >70 g/L and thus a red cell transfusion can be avoided at this point.

As her anaemia has developed secondary to low iron stores, the patient should be treated with iron therapy, either orally or intravenously. An intravenous iron infusion is more appropriate in this case, to ensure that the iron stores are corrected rapidly, as the patient has symptoms of light-headedness. Intravenous iron therapy results in higher haemoglobin levels and a reduced need for red cell transfusions compared to oral iron replacement.

The patient's general practitioner should subsequently re-check her full blood count and haematinics and consider prescribing oral iron replacement if needed.

History
A 72-year-old man presented to his GP complaining of constipation. He reported increasing difficulty opening his bowels for 3 weeks. He was passing small lumps of hard brown stool every 1–2 days. There was no blood or mucus present, and he had no problems with his bowels prior to this. He underwent a medication review 4 weeks earlier and attributed his new symptoms to the prescription changes that were made. He denied experiencing weight loss, back pain or abdominal pain.

Examination
Systems examination identified a soft but slightly distended abdomen with no tenderness on palpation. Digital rectal examination found impacted hard brown stool in the rectum.

Question
Of the medications below, which *two* are known to commonly cause constipation?

Amitriptyline	☐
Amoxicillin	☐
Paracetamol	☐
Verapamil	☐
Warfarin	☐

ANSWER

Amitriptyline	X
Amoxicillin	☐
Paracetamol	☐
Verapamil	X
Warfarin	☐

Nausea, diarrhoea and constipation are among the most frequently reported adverse drug reactions. The association between opioids and constipation is well-known, but it is important to advise patients that they may experience a change in bowel habit when starting other medications too.

Calcium channel antagonists, particularly verapamil, are associated with reduced gastro-intestinal motility. Both the tricyclic and selective serotonin reuptake inhibitor antidepressants and anti-cholinergic drugs such as diphenhydramine and oxybutynin can also slow gut transit.

History

A 75-year-old man has been admitted to hospital with shortness of breath and a wheeze. He is diagnosed with an infective exacerbation of chronic obstructive pulmonary disease and is treated with a course of amoxicillin 500 mg IV TDS, prednisolone 30 mg PO OD, and salbutamol and ipratropium bromide nebulisers. Shortly after his hospital admission, the patient is noted to have impaired swallowing function and is advised to be 'nil-by-mouth' until a nasogastric tube is sited.

Question

You are asked to convert the patient's oral corticosteroids to an equivalent dose of intravenous hydrocortisone. Using the drug chart below, please prescribe an intravenous alternative.

DRUG (print approved name)		Dose	Date					
			6					
			8					
Signature	Date	Route	12					
Print name	Bleep	Pharmacy	14					
			18					
Additional information			22					

ANSWER

Prednisolone 30 mg is equivalent to hydrocortisone 120 mg.

DRUG (print approved name)		Dose	Date						
			6						
HYDROCORTISONE		120 mg	(8)						
Signature *A Doctor*	Date 01/01/20	Route IV	12						
Print name A DOCTOR	Bleep 1234	Pharmacy	14						
			18						
Additional information 5 day course, IECOPD			22						

There are many resources available to facilitate the conversion of one corticosteroid to an equivalent dose (based on anti-inflammatory potency) of another corticosteroid. The British National Formulary, for example, includes a table containing this data.

Equivalent doses of prednisolone are shown below:

Prednisolone 5 mg is equivalent to:	Dexamethasone 750 mg Hydrocortisone 20 mg Methylprednisolone 4 mg

History
A 26-year-old woman presents to the emergency department complaining of palpitations. She has been feeling hot and tremulous for the past week and has noticed that she is sweating excessively. She has no past medical history, has no known drug allergies and takes no regular medications. She works as an actress, does not drink alcohol, does not smoke and does not take recreational drugs.

Examination
The patient was afebrile and appeared clinically well. Her heart rate was 120 bpm and her blood pressure was 126/80 mmHg. Her abdomen was soft and non-tender. She had a fine tremor.

Results
ECG: sinus tachycardia, HR 110

Bloods: WCC 9.2, Hb 140, Plt 374, Na 138, K 4.1, Creat 70, CRP <1, TSH <0.1 mIU/L

Question
Based on the above information, the patient is advised to commence treatment for hyperthyroidism with carbimazole. Select the *two* most appropriate statements below that should be explained to the patient regarding carbimazole therapy.

She should discuss any symptoms suggestive of infection, such as a sore throat, with a medical practitioner	☐
She can continue to donate blood every 3–4 months whilst on carbimazole therapy	☐
Her symptoms of palpitations and tremor will resolve immediately after commencing carbimazole therapy	☐
She should not drink alcohol whilst on carbimazole therapy	☐
She must use effective contraception during treatment with carbimazole	☐

ANSWER

She should discuss any symptoms suggestive of infection, such as a sore throat, with a medical practitioner	X
She can continue to donate blood every 3–4 months whilst on carbimazole therapy	☐
Her symptoms of palpitations and tremor will resolve immediately after commencing carbimazole therapy	☐
She should not drink alcohol whilst on carbimazole therapy	☐
She must use effective contraception during treatment with carbimazole	X

Carbimazole reduces the production of the thyroid hormones T_3 and T_4 (thyroxine) and is thus used in the treatment of hyperthyroidism. One of the recognised adverse effects of carbimazole is bone marrow suppression and the subsequent development of neutropaenia and agranulocytosis. Patients should be advised to discuss symptoms such as mouth ulcers developing, a sore throat, fevers, bruising easily and any signs or symptoms of an infection with a medical practitioner. A full blood count will then be taken to identify potential bone marrow suppression.

Carbimazole use is associated with the development of congenital malformations and women of childbearing potential should ensure that they are using effective contraception. Contraception that is considered to be 'highly effective' has a <1% failure rate and includes: an intrauterine device (IUD), an intrauterine system (IUS), the progestogen-only implant and sterilisation.

Patients should not donate blood whilst taking carbimazole and for a further 24 months after completing carbimazole therapy.

Patients should also be informed that their symptoms of hyperthyroidism are unlikely to resolve within the first 2 weeks of carbimazole therapy, and that it may take up to 2 months for full symptom resolution.

Question

Of these antiplatelet agents, identify the *two* that have dosage errors:

Aspirin	75 mg	PO	OD	☐
Cilostazol	100 mg	PO	BD	☐
Clopidogrel	7.5 mg	PO	OD	☐
Dipyridamole (modified release)	200 mg	PO	BD	☐
Prasugrel	10 mg	PO	OD	☐
Ticagrelor	90 mg	PO	OD	☐

ANSWER

Aspirin	75 mg	PO	OD	☐
Cilostazol	100 mg	PO	BD	☐
Clopidogrel	7.5 mg	PO	OD	X
Dipyridamole (modified release)	200 mg	PO	BD	☐
Prasugrel	10 mg	PO	OD	☐
Ticagrelor	90 mg	PO	OD	X

Clopidogrel should be prescribed as a 75 mg PO OD dose – not 7.5 mg PO OD. Always ensure that the decimal points are in the correct place and that the units are also correct when prescribing medications.

Ticagrelor is an ADP antagonist that reversibly inhibits the $P2Y_{12}$ receptor. Ticagrelor is prescribed twice daily rather than once daily.

History

A 53-year-old woman was brought to hospital complaining of chest pain. The pain was described as crushing in nature and was located over the centre of her chest, radiating to the left arm and jaw. She felt nauseated but had not vomited. Her past medical history included hypertension and type 2 diabetes mellitus. Her regular medications were: amlodipine 10 mg OD, ramipril 5 mg OD, metformin 1 g BD and gliclazide 80 mg OD.

Examination

The patient was distressed but alert and orientated. Her heart sounds were dual with no murmurs. Her heart rate was 75 bpm and her blood pressure was 150/96 mmHg. Her chest was clear, her respiratory rate was 20 and her peripheral oxygen saturations were 96% on room air. There was no peripheral oedema.

Results

Bloods: Na 142, K 4.6, Creat 80, Mg 0.86, TnT 50

ECG: see below

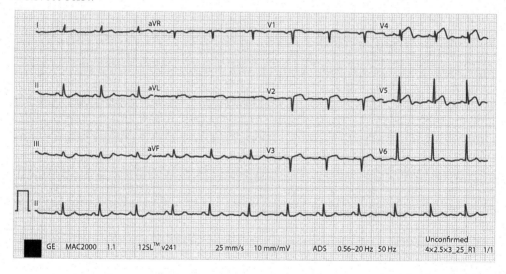

Case progression

The patient was diagnosed with an ST-elevation myocardial infarction and underwent successful percutaneous coronary intervention. Several hours later, she was transferred to the coronary care unit. On arrival the nurse noted that the patient's heart rate had risen to 200 bpm. There was no clinical deterioration – the patient remained alert and orientated and did not report any further chest pain. Her blood pressure was 105/72 mmHg.

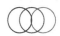

A repeat ECG strip, printed from the defibrillator, is shown below:

Delayed

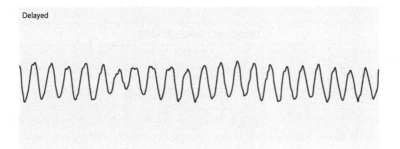

Question

In view of the findings on the above ECG strip, please prescribe the most appropriate *one* medication to be given at this point.

ONCE ONLY MEDICATIONS									
Date	Medication	Dose	Route	Time of dose	Signature	Prescriber	Given by	Time given	Pharmacy

ANSWER

ONCE ONLY MEDICATIONS									
Date	Medication	Dose	Route	Time of dose	Signature	Prescriber	Given by	Time given	Pharmacy
01/01/20	AMIODARONE	300 mg	IV	12:00	*A Doctor*	A DOCTOR			

The rhythm strip shows a broad complex tachycardia consistent with ventricular tachycardia. The priority at this moment is to administer amiodarone 300 mg IV, ideally through a large bore cannula or a central line. This should be delivered over 20–60 min. Once the infusion is completed, a further amiodarone infusion of 900 mg over 24 h should then be commenced.

The patient has no obvious electrolyte abnormalities to correct but may nevertheless benefit from an intravenous infusion of magnesium as higher serum concentrations of magnesium reduce the risk of arrhythmias developing.

CASE 80: DRUG MONITORING 6

History

A 42-year-old man undergoes a renal transplant and subsequently commences treatment with oral tacrolimus 12 h post-transplant. You are asked to discuss tacrolimus therapy with the patient.

Question

Which *two* of the following statements regarding tacrolimus monitoring is correct?

Tacrolimus levels do not need to be monitored in patients with normal renal function post-transplant	☐
If tacrolimus levels are too high, the eGFR may decline	☐
If tacrolimus levels are too low, the eGFR may decline	☐
If tacrolimus levels are too low, the patient may develop signs of drug toxicity	☐
Patients using topical tacrolimus will never need to have tacrolimus levels measured	☐

ANSWER

Tacrolimus levels do not need to be monitored in patients with normal renal function post-transplant	☐
If tacrolimus levels are too high, the eGFR may decline	X
If tacrolimus levels are too low, the eGFR may decline	X
If tacrolimus levels are too low, the patient may develop signs of toxicity	☐
Patients using topical tacrolimus will never need to have tacrolimus levels measured	☐

Tacrolimus is a calcineurin inhibitor with immunosuppressive properties, and is commonly used following hepatic or renal transplants to prevent graft rejection. Tacrolimus has a narrow therapeutic index and levels should be regularly checked in patients who take this medication.

Elevated tacrolimus levels increase the risk of developing tacrolimus toxicity, which can manifest with a variety of signs, including nephrotoxicity and neurotoxicity. Low tacrolimus levels indicate inadequate immunosuppression, meaning the graft may begin to fail. In both situations, the patient's renal function may deteriorate and the tacrolimus level can help in identifying the cause.

Tacrolimus can also be used topically to treat a variety of dermatological conditions, including severe atopic eczema. Tacrolimus levels are typically not required; however, in some situations where the skin barrier is not intact, significant percutaneous absorption may occur and tacrolimus levels may be measured to assess for tacrolimus toxicity.

History
A 74-year-old man was admitted to hospital complaining of diarrhoea. He reported passing watery green-brown stool, up to 20 times in the preceding 24 h. He had not experienced any episodes of vomiting or abdominal pain. His past medical history included chronic obstructive pulmonary disease, with several infective exacerbations over the past 2 months, all of which were treated with courses of prednisolone and antibiotics. His regular medications included carbocisteine 375 mg BD, a salbutamol inhaler and a budesonide/formoterol combination inhaler. He was a retired psychologist, was an ex-smoker with a 40-pack year history, and did not drink alcohol regularly.

Examination
The patient was febrile (temperature 38.0°C), tachycardic (HR 100) and hypotensive (BP 96/68 mmHg). His abdomen was soft but distended and his bowel sounds were high pitched.

Results
Bloods: WCC 28.4, Hb 130, Plt 409, Na 133, K 3.2, Creat 98, CRP 88

Stool culture: *Clostridium difficile* bacteria identified

Abdominal X-ray: see below

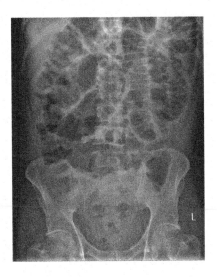

Question
Which *one* of the below therapies would be most appropriate for this patient?

Amoxicillin-clavulanate (co-amoxiclav)	1.2 g	IV	TDS	☐
Doxycycline	200 mg	PO	OD	☐
Flucloxacillin	1 g	IV	QDS	☐
Gentamicin	80 mg	IV	OD	☐
Vancomycin	125 mg	PO	QDS	☐

ANSWER

Amoxicillin-clavulanate (co-amoxiclav)	1.2 g	IV	TDS	☐
Doxycycline	200 mg	PO	OD	☐
Flucloxacillin	1 g	IV	QDS	☐
Gentamicin	80 mg	IV	OD	☐
Vancomycin	125 mg	PO	QDS	X

The patient's symptoms are consistent with a gastrointestinal infection. His blood results show elevated inflammatory markers (a very elevated leucocytosis is typical for moderate-severe *Clostridium difficile* infections). His stool cultures have grown *Clostridium difficile* bacteria and his abdominal X-ray shows prominent dilated loops of bowel.

This patient has received multiple doses of antibiotics over recent months, which may have contributed to the development of *Clostridium difficile* infection. Antibiotics can disrupt the usual gut flora leading to diarrhoea, in some cases, increased replication of particular bacteria, including *Clostridium difficile*. Antibiotic-associated diarrhoea is more likely to develop following administration of clindamycin, cephalosporins, amoxicillin-clavulanate (co-amoxiclav) and quinolones.

Very mild cases of *Clostridium difficile* colitis can be observed without treatment for 48–72 h. Several antibiotics can be used to treat *Clostridium difficile* infections, including oral metro-nidazole 500 mg TDS, for mild/moderate disease.

First-line treatment for moderate-severe *Clostridium difficile* infections is oral vancomycin. Fidaxomicin is typically reserved for second-line therapy or when intravenous treatment is preferred.

History

A 90-year-old man is brought to hospital by his son who has become concerned that his father is intermittently drowsy and difficult to rouse. He has noticed his father falling asleep during conversations and he has spilt hot drinks over himself on several occasions. The patient agrees that he has experienced excessive somnolence over recent weeks and he attributes this to a change in his medications one month earlier. The patient is unsure of his regular medications but denies having any allergies. He lives alone, does not drink alcohol and is an ex-smoker with a 30-pack year history.

Examination

Systems examination, including a full neurological examination, was unremarkable.

Results

An arterial blood gas performed on room air showed normal gas exchange and acid-base balance.

Question

Of the medications below, which two are known to commonly cause increased drowsiness?

Alendronic acid	☐
Aspirin	☐
Carbocisteine	☐
Chlordiazepoxide	☐
Diphenhydramine	☐
Omeprazole	☐
Paracetamol	☐

ANSWER

Alendronic acid	☐
Aspirin	☐
Carbocisteine	☐
Chlordiazepoxide	X
Diphenhydramine	X
Omeprazole	☐
Paracetamol	☐

Many medications can cause fatigue or drowsiness, particularly in elderly patients. Drowsiness is a common adverse effect of both opioids and benzodiazepines (of which chlordiazepoxide is one). Chlordiazepoxide is prescribed to manage anxiety in some patients, and is frequently used to manage alcohol withdrawal symptoms in the hospital inpatient setting.

Antihistamines, particularly first-generation antihistamines such as diphenhydramine, are lipid soluble, and cross the blood–brain barrier where they inhibit central H_1 receptor activity – this results in central nervous system adverse effects, including drowsiness.

Other drugs that can cause fatigue include anti-hypertensives, particularly drugs that reduce the cardiac output, such as beta-receptor blockers (e.g. bisoprolol).

History
A 70-year-old man was admitted to hospital with shortness of breath, severe lower back pain and general decline. During his hospital stay, he was diagnosed with lung cancer with widespread metastases, including spinal deposits. He became increasingly drowsy and the palliative care team advised that the patient should be prescribed subcutaneous medications to control any symptoms that should arise.

Question
The patient had been taking morphine immediate release solution 5 mg PO up to 4 hourly, as required. Using the chart below, please prescribe an equivalent dose of subcutaneous morphine.

DRUG (print approved name)		Dose	Date					
			Time					
Signature	Date	Route	Dose					
Print name	Bleep	Pharmacy	Route					
Indication/additional information		Max dose freq	Name					

ANSWER

Morphine immediate release solution 5 mg PO up to 4 hourly is equivalent to morphine 2.5 mg SC up to 4 hourly.

DRUG (print approved name) MORPHINE		Dose 2.5 mg	Date							
			Time							
Signature *a DOCTOR*	Date 01/01/20	Route SC	Dose							
Print name A DOCTOR	Bleep 1234	Pharmacy	Route							
Indication/additional information FOR PAIN		Max dose freq 4 HOURLY	Name							

There are many resources available to facilitate the conversion of one opioid analgesic to either an equivalent dose in an alternative formulation or to another opioid analgesic. The British National Formulary, for example, includes a table containing this data.

Morphine 10 mg PO is equivalent to:	Codeine phosphate/dihydrocodeine 100 mg PO
	Morphine 5 mg IV/IM/SC
	Oxycodone 6.6 mg PO

History

A 16-year-old woman presented to her family planning centre to ask for advice. She had been taking the combined oral contraceptive pill (Cilest®) for the past 6 months but missed her last two doses of this. She was currently taking the second week of her pill pack and had had unprotected vaginal intercourse within the last 24 h.

She had no past medical history and took no other medications regularly. She was a school student and did not drink alcohol or smoke cigarettes.

Results

A urine pregnancy test was negative for β-HCG.

Question

Based on the above information, select the two most appropriate statements below that should be explained to the patient.

She should take the last pill that she missed now, even if this means taking two pills in 1 day	☐
She should wait until the next pill is due and then continue taking the pill daily	☐
She will be offered emergency contraception to prevent pregnancy	☐
She should use extra contraception, such as condoms, for the next 7 days	☐
She will not need to use extra contraception to prevent pregnancy	☐

ANSWER

She should take the last pill that she missed now, even if this means taking two pills in 1 day	X
She should wait until the next pill is due and then continue taking the pill daily	☐
She will be offered emergency contraception to prevent pregnancy	☐
She should use extra contraception, such as condoms, for the next 7 days	X
She will not need to use extra contraception to prevent pregnancy	☐

The combined oral contraceptive pill is more than 99% effective at preventing pregnancy if used correctly. If one pill is missed at any point in the pack or a new pack is started 1 day late, patients are still effectively protected against pregnancy. They should take the pill that they missed as soon as possible, even if this means taking two pills in 1 day.

If two or more pills are missed, the patient should take the last pill that they missed as soon as possible, even if this means taking two pills in 1 day and use extra contraception, such as condoms, during vaginal intercourse for the next 7 days. If the pills were missed in the first week of the pill pack, emergency contraception should be considered to prevent pregnancy.

History

A 24-year-old man presented to the emergency room after developing palpitations. He reported that he had attended a party the night before where he had consumed 12–14 pints of beer. When he awoke the following morning, he was aware of palpitations but had not experienced chest pain or shortness of breath. He had no significant past medical history and did not take any medications. He worked in digital marketing as a social media influencer, smoked approximately 10 cigarettes per week and drank approximately 25 units of alcohol per week. He denied any recreational drug use.

Examination

The patient appeared clinically well. His heart rate was 170 and his blood pressure was 140/80 mmHg.

Results

Bloods: WCC 5.1, Hb 162, Plt 320, Na 138, K 4.0, Creat 76, Mg 0.90, CRP <1

ECG: see below

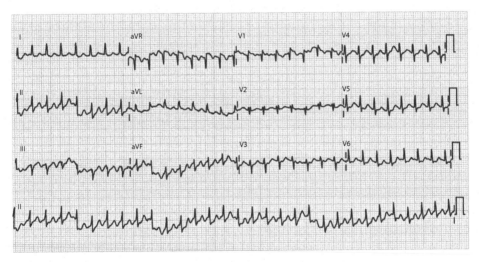

Question

Based on the above information, prescribe the most appropriate treatment for this patient.

ONCE ONLY MEDICATIONS									
Date	Medication	Dose	Route	Time of dose	Signature	Prescriber	Given by	Time given	Pharmacy

ANSWER

ONCE ONLY MEDICATIONS									
Date	Medication	Dose	Route	Time of dose	Signature	Prescriber	Given by	Time given	Pharmacy
01/01/20	ADENOSINE	6 mg	IV	12:00	*a Doctor*	A DOCTOR			

The patient's ECG shows a narrow complex tachycardia consistent with supraventricular tachycardia (SVT). The appropriate treatment for this in a conscious, haemodynamically stable patient is an intravenous bolus of adenosine 6 mg (ideally pushed in rapidly via a large-bore cannula and then flushed with 20 mL 0.9% sodium chloride).

If the SVT persists or the patient cardioverts and then reverts back to SVT, two further 12 mg doses of adenosine can be given.

History

A 56-year-old man was admitted to hospital complaining of severe chest pain. The pain was located over the centre of his chest, was crushing in nature, 10/10 in severity and radiated to his left arm and jaw. His past medical history included hypertension, type 2 diabetes mellitus and angina pectoris. His regular medications included: aspirin 75 mg OD, ramipril 5 mg OD, metformin 1 g BD and atorvastatin 20 mg ON. He worked as an office manager, smoked 20 cigarettes daily and drank 30 units of alcohol per week.

Question

You are asked to prescribe an intravenous glyceryl trinitrate (GTN) infusion to relieve the patient's chest pain. What *two* factors should guide the titration of this infusion?

The patient's systolic blood pressure	☐
The patient's heart rate	☐
The patient's pain	☐
The patient's brain natriuretic peptide level	☐
The patient's serum troponin level	☐

100 Cases in Clinical Pharmacology, Therapeutics and Prescribing

ANSWER

The patient's systolic blood pressure	X
The patient's heart rate	☐
The patient's pain	X
The patient's brain natriuretic peptide level	☐
The patient's serum troponin level	☐

A GTN infusion may be prescribed for patients who have developed pulmonary oedema or those with ongoing ischaemic cardiac pain that does not resolve with either sublingual GTN or intravenous morphine.

GTN is a 'nitric oxide donor' and increases vasodilation. As a result, coronary blood flow increases. Hypotension is a common adverse event associated with GTN administration.

The patient's pain and their systolic blood pressure should be used to guide titration of the infusion rate every 15–30 min, with the initial rate starting at 1 mg/h and potentially being increased to 10 mg/h.

History
A 28-year-old woman presented to hospital with a 12-h history of progressive shortness of breath and left-sided chest pain. The chest pain was exacerbated by deep inspiration and coughing. Her past medical history included a deep vein thrombosis in her right calf 3 years earlier and two miscarriages in the third trimester of pregnancy. She took no regular medications and had no known drug allergies. She worked as a traffic warden, did not smoke, and drank around 10 units of alcohol per week.

Examination
The patient appeared dyspnoeic but otherwise well. Her heart rate was 80 bpm and her blood pressure was 124/90 mmHg. Her heart sounds were normal. Her chest was clear, her respiratory rate was 18 and her peripheral oxygen saturations (SpO$_2$) were 97% on room air.

Results
Bloods: WCC 10.1, Hb 135, Plt 280

CT pulmonary angiogram: there is a left-sided subsegmental pulmonary embolus

Progress
The patient was advised that she was likely to have an underlying prothrombotic condition, such as antiphospholipid syndrome, based on her history of recurrent venous thromboemboli.

Question
Which *one* of the treatments below is most appropriate for this patient to be discharged home with?

Apixaban	10 mg	PO	BD	☐
Aspirin	75 mg	PO	OD	☐
Compression stockings	1 pair	TOP	OD	☐
Rivaroxaban	15 mg	PO	BD	☐
Warfarin	7 mg	PO	OD	☐

ANSWER

Apixaban	10 mg	PO	BD	☐
Aspirin	75 mg	PO	OD	☐
Compression stockings	1 pair	TOP	OD	☐
Rivaroxaban	15 mg	PO	BD	☐
Warfarin	7 mg	PO	OD	X

Although it has not yet been proven, there is a high likelihood that the patient has a pro-thrombotic condition, such as antiphospholipid disease, based on her history of recurrent venous thromboembolism and multiple miscarriages.

Patients with deep vein thromboses and pulmonary emboli are now commonly treated with a direct oral anticoagulant, such as rivaroxaban or apixaban. In this case, where the patient has suspected antiphospholipid syndrome, commencing lifelong anticoagulation with warfarin is the correct answer. Currently, direct oral anticoagulants are not used in patients with antiphospholipid syndrome as recent studies have shown that they are inferior in preventing venous thromboembolism compared to warfarin.

History

A 62-year-old man presented to the emergency department complaining of a painful left knee. He reported that the pain developed 3 days earlier and had gradually progressed. He had not experienced swelling of any other joints and had been generally well with no fevers or recent illnesses. He had not experienced any trauma. His past medical history included hypertension and gastro-oesophageal reflux disease. He was unable to recall his regular medications. He worked as a shop manager and did not drink alcohol regularly. He had never smoked.

Examination

The patient had a swollen left knee with a large effusion overlying the joint space.

Results

Synovial fluid aspiration: needle-shaped negatively birefringent crystals, consistent with a diagnosis of gout

Questions

1. Which *two* medications could be initiated to treat the acute flare of gout?
2. Long-term use of which *one* medication is most strongly associated with acute flares of gout?

	1	2
Allopurinol	☐	☐
Amlodipine	☐	☐
Bendroflumethiazide	☐	☐
Colchicine	☐	☐
Dihydrocodeine	☐	☐
Ibuprofen	☐	☐
Omeprazole	☐	☐
Paracetamol	☐	☐

ANSWERS

	1	2
Allopurinol	□	□
Amlodipine	□	□
Bendroflumethiazide	□	X
Colchicine	X	□
Dihydrocodeine	□	□
Ibuprofen	X	□
Omeprazole	□	□
Paracetamol	□	□

1. Gout is a condition where elevated uric acid concentrations results in the formation and deposition of urate crystals in one or more joints. An acute flare of gout can occur following multiple triggers including an injury to the joint, alcohol excess or stress. Patients may develop chronic gout over a number of years, with intermittent episodes where the symptoms flare up acutely.

    Acute flares of gout are treated with non-steroidal anti-inflammatory drugs (NSAIDs), to reduce inflammation around the affected joint(s). Colchicine is an alkaloid that is also used to treat acute flares of gout. The exact mechanism of colchicine in treating gout flares is unclear although it appears to interrupt the cycle of urate crystal deposition within joints.

    Allopurinol is a xanthine oxidase inhibitor that reduces uric acid production. Allopurinol and other urate lowering therapies are traditionally commenced 2–4 weeks after an acute flare of gout as the reduction in uric acid levels may cause urate crystals to be shed into the joint space, worsening the inflammation within the joint.

2. Certain medications can increase uric acid concentrations, increasing the risk of developing gout. Loop and thiazide diuretics, for example, increase uric acid reabsorption resulting in higher serum uric acid levels.

History

A 40-year-old woman is admitted to hospital complaining of a painful, swollen right calf. The patient had recently travelled from Sydney to London, which involved more than 28 h of travelling. She was otherwise well, with no known additional risk factors for developing a venous thromboembolism.

Examination

The patient's right calf appeared swollen and erythematous. Systems examination was otherwise unremarkable.

Results

Bloods: WCC 8.7, Hb 134, Plt 450, Na 138, K 3.6, Creat 52 (eGFR 120)

Doppler ultrasound scan: in the right lower limb there is visible thrombus extending into the popliteal vein

Question

You have been asked to prescribe subcutaneous enoxaparin, a form of low molecular weight heparin.

The patient weighs 60 kg.

Using information from the British National Formulary, an equivalent resource or local guidelines, please calculate the dose of enoxaparin that should be prescribed to treat this patient's deep vein thrombosis.

The patient should be given a dose of enoxaparin [   ] mg SC.

ANSWER

Enoxaparin is prescribed at a dose of 1.5 mg/kg in patients with a venous thromboembolism. This is assuming that they have normal renal function and do not have additional risk factors for developing a venous thromboembolism.

This patient weighs 60 kg, so she should be prescribed enoxaparin 90 mg SC every 24 h.

History

A 27-year-old man presented to the emergency department complaining of abdominal pain and diarrhoea. The abdominal pain was cramping in nature and was relieved by opening his bowels. His stools were watery brown with small amounts of fresh blood mixed in. He was passing stool up to 20 times per day and was waking overnight to open his bowels. His past medical history included ulcerative colitis, which had been diagnosed 9 months earlier. He was not currently taking any regular medications. He worked as a solicitor, drank 20 units of alcohol per week and had never smoked.

Examination

The patient was afebrile. His heart rate was 90 bpm and his blood pressure was 128/86 mmHg. The patient's abdomen was tender over the left iliac fossa but was soft throughout with hyperactive bowel sounds. On digital examination, the rectum was empty.

Results

Bloods: WCC 12.9, Hb 108, Plt 389, Na 135, K 3.5, Creat 78, CRP 120

Abdominal X-ray: unremarkable, no bowel dilation seen

Question

The patient was diagnosed with a flare of ulcerative colitis. Which *two* of the following treatment options would be most appropriate in this case?

Low molecular weight heparin should be prescribed as venous thromboembolism prophylaxis	☐
Low molecular weight heparin should not be prescribed as the patient has rectal bleeding	☐
Loperamide should be prescribed to reduce the frequency of bowel motions	☐
Prednisolone 30 mg PO OD should be commenced to reduce the inflammatory response	☐
Hydrocortisone 100 mg IV QDS should be commenced to reduce the inflammatory response	☐

ANSWER

Low molecular weight heparin should be prescribed as venous thromboembolism prophylaxis	X
Low molecular weight heparin should not be prescribed as the patient has rectal bleeding	☐
Loperamide should be prescribed to reduce the frequency of bowel motions	☐
Prednisolone 30 mg PO OD should be commenced to reduce the inflammatory response	☐
Hydrocortisone 100 mg IV QDS should be commenced to reduce the inflammatory response	X

This patient meets the criteria of acute moderate to severe ulcerative colitis and should be treated with intravenous corticosteroids; hydrocortisone or methylprednisolone would be appropriate. The patient should also be referred to the on-call surgical team who will assess the need for surgical intervention.

Loperamide should not be prescribed routinely in acute ulcerative colitis as this can increase the risk of developing bowel dilatation and toxic megacolon.

A flare of ulcerative colitis is a pro-thrombotic state and patients with either no rectal bleeding or non-severe rectal bleeding (not requiring red cell transfusion or resulting in haemodynamic instability) should be prescribed venous thromboprophylaxis with low molecular weight heparin.

History

A 58-year-old man presented to his general practitioner complaining of shortness of breath. He reported a 12-month history of difficulty expectorating and reported that his sputum was extremely thick and sticky. He had received multiple courses of antibiotics and steroids in the past few months with no subsequent improvement in his symptoms. He had otherwise been well over recent weeks. His past medical history included chronic obstructive pulmonary disease. His regular medications were: (i) a Trimbow® combination inhaler (containing beclomethasone, formoterol and glycopyrronium) two puffs twice daily and (ii) a salbutamol 200 µg inhaler two puffs as required. He worked as a pub landlord and drank approximately 20 units of alcohol per week and was a current smoker of 20 cigarettes daily.

Examination

The patient was afebrile. His respiratory rate was 18 and his peripheral oxygen saturations were 96% on room air. There was a mild expiratory wheeze heard throughout the chest.

Question

Prescribe a drug to reduce this patient's sputum viscosity using the chart below.

		Date					
DRUG (print approved name)	Dose	6					
		8					
Signature / Date	Route	12					
Print name / Bleep	Pharmacy	14					
		18					
Additional information		22					

ANSWER

		Date						
DRUG (print approved name)	Dose	6						
CARBOCISTEINE	750 mg	(8)						
Signature	Date	Route	12					
A Doctor	01/01/20	PO						
Print name	Bleep	Pharmacy	(14)					
A DOCTOR	1234		18					
Additional information								
PCP prophylaxis			(22)					

Carbocisteine should initially be prescribed at a dose of 2.25 g daily in divided doses, then reduced to 1.5 g daily in divided doses once the symptoms improve. Carbocisteine is a mucolytic drug that acts by modulating metabolism of mucus producing cells. Patients taking mucolytics develop thinner respiratory secretions that are easier to expectorate. This may reduce exacerbations of chronic obstructive pulmonary disease in some patients. Alternative mucolytics include acetylcysteine, which acts by hydrolysing disulphide bonds in mucins, and erdosteine, which increases mucociliary transport.

History

A 64-year-old woman presented to her general practitioner complaining of a painful genitals. She reported a 4-day history of discomfort and pruritus around her vulva and was struggling to pass urine due to the pain. Her past medical history included polymyalgia rheumatica and her current medications were ibuprofen 400 mg PO TDS and prednisolone 20 mg PO OD. She had no known drug allergies and worked as a headmistress. She did not drink alcohol regularly or smoke.

Examination

The vulva appeared erythematous and swollen. White vaginal discharge was present. Systems examination was otherwise unremarkable.

Results

Vaginal swab result: heavy growth of *Candida albicans*

Question

Based on the above medication, which *two* treatments would be most appropriate for the patient?

Amoxicillin (1 dose)	500 mg	PO	☐
Amphoterecin (1 dose)	5 mg/kg	OD	☐
Clotrimazole (pessary, 1 dose)	500 mg	PV	☐
Flucloxacillin (1 dose)	500 mg	PO	☐
Fluconazole (1 dose)	150 mg	PO	☐

ANSWER

Amoxicillin (1 dose)	500 mg	PO	☐
Amphoterecin (1 dose)	5 mg/kg	OD	☐
Clotrimazole (pessary, 1 dose)	500 mg	PV	X
Flucloxacillin (1 dose)	500 mg	PO	☐
Fluconazole (1 dose)	150 mg	PO	X

The patient has vaginal candidiasis, often referred to as 'thrush'. This is a common infection that 75% of women will experience at least once in their lifetime. Generally, no obvious cause is identified; however, precipitants can include corticosteroid use (this patient is currently taking a course of prednisolone), diabetes mellitus and other causes of immunosuppression.

Any patient with recurrent candidiasis (>1 episode per 6 months) should have a HbA1c test to assess their glycaemic control.

The infection can be treated with a variety of anti-fungal therapies, including clotrimazole pessaries, with clotrimazole vaginal creams, or a one-off dose of a fluconazole tablet – most women favour the oral therapy, with vaginal creams to reduce local irritation if needed.

History

A 77-year-old man was brought to hospital after collapsing on the bus. He reported standing up when the bus reached his stop and suddenly finding himself lying on the floor. He described feeling light-headed and as though his vision were 'blacking out' in the seconds preceding his collapse. Eye witnesses reported that he lost consciousness for several seconds and subsequently awoke and was fully orientated. There was no tongue biting, jerking of limbs or incontinence. The patient denied experiencing any chest pain, shortness of breath or palpitations prior to the collapse. He had experienced several similar episodes of collapse after standing recently. The patient's past medical history included benign prostatic hyperplasia, ischaemic heart disease and type 2 diabetes mellitus. His regular medications are listed below. The patient owned and worked on a local market stall every day selling fruit and vegetables. He did not drink alcohol and was a current smoker of 20 cigarettes daily, with a 50-pack year history.

Examination

The patient appeared clinically well. His heart rate was 70 bpm and his blood pressure when lying down was 130/84 mmHg. His blood pressure fell to 86/60 mmHg on standing. His chest was clear, his oxygen saturations were 97% on room air and his abdomen was soft and non-tender. Neurological examination was unremarkable.

Results

Bloods: WCC 10.0, Hb 130, Plt 336, Na 137, K 3.5, Creat 62, glucose 6.4

ECG: normal sinus rhythm

Question

Which *two* of the following medications may have caused the patient to collapse?

Aspirin	75 mg	PO	OD	☐
Atorvastatin	40 mg	PO	ON	☐
Calcium carbonate/vitamin D_3	2 × 750 mg/200 I.U.	PO	BD	☐
Isosorbide mononitrate	40 mg	PO	BD	☐
Metformin	500 mg	PO	BD	☐
Ranitidine	150 mg	PO	BD	☐
Tamsulosin (modified release)	400 mg	PO	OD	☐

ANSWER

Aspirin	75 mg	PO	OD	☐
Atorvastatin	40 mg	PO	ON	☐
Calcium carbonate/vitamin D_3	2 × 750 mg/200 I.U.	PO	BD	☐
Isosorbide mononitrate	40 mg	PO	BD	X
Metformin	500 mg	PO	BD	☐
Ranitidine	150 mg	PO	BD	☐
Tamsulosin (modified release)	400 mg	PO	OD	X

The symptoms preceding the patient's collapse (feeling light headed on standing, his vision fading to black) is in keeping with syncope. He has a marked postural drop, making orthostatic hypotension a likely cause for the syncopal episode.

Most antihypertensive agents can cause a degree of orthostatic postural hypotension; however, the administration of alpha receptor blockers (e.g. doxazosin) or nitrate-based drugs (e.g. isosorbide mononitrate) is considerably more likely to result in a significant postural drop. Symptoms are often more prominent after the first dose of the medication ('first-dose hypotension'). Tamsulosin is an alpha receptor blocker that is used in the treatment of benign prostatic hyperplasia.

History

A 17-year-old woman called her general practitioner to ask for telephone advice regarding her blood glucose management. She had been feeling unwell for the past 2 days with a flu-like illness and had experienced a significant reduction in her appetite and, consequently, her oral intake. Her main complaints were of a dry cough, feeling feverish and coryzal symptoms. The patient's past medical history included type 1 diabetes mellitus and she used a long-acting insulin, plus boluses of a short-acting insulin to manage her glycaemic control. She was working as an apprentice in mechanics and did not drink alcohol or smoke cigarettes.

Question

Based on the above information, select the *two* most appropriate statements below that should be explained to the patient regarding her glycaemic control.

The patient should continue using her regular insulin doses and seek further advice	☐
The patient should increase her regular insulin doses and seek further advice if she becomes more unwell	☐
The patient should reduce her regular insulin doses and seek further advice if she becomes more unwell	☐
The patient should continue monitoring her blood glucose levels as normal	☐
The patient should increase the frequency at which she checks her blood glucose levels	☐

ANSWER

The patient should continue using her regular insulin doses and seek further advice	X
The patient should increase her regular insulin doses and seek further advice if she becomes more unwell	☐
The patient should reduce her regular insulin doses and seek further advice if she becomes more unwell	☐
The patient should continue monitoring her blood glucose levels as normal	☐
The patient should increase the frequency at which she checks her blood glucose levels	X

The patient is likely to have a viral upper respiratory tract infection and currently sounds relatively well. Patients who have an acute illness but are not vomiting should be advised to continue their regular insulin treatment, even if their oral intake is reduced, as glucose levels often rise in illness as part of the stress response.

The patient should be advised to ensure that she is well-hydrated and to monitor her blood glucose levels more frequently. She should also check for the presence of ketones in her blood.

The patient should attend her local emergency department if she begins vomiting, if her blood glucose levels rise above 15 mmol/L, or if she develops ketones in her blood as she will be at risk of developing diabetic ketoacidosis.

CASE 95: PROVIDING INFORMATION 7

History

A 55-year-old man presented to the emergency department complaining of palpitations and shortness of breath. He felt the palpitations developed suddenly 45 min earlier. He had been unwell with diarrhoea and vomiting over the preceding 2 days, as had other members of the household. His past medical history included ischaemic heart disease and a previous myocardial infarction 4 years earlier, for which he underwent a percutaneous coronary intervention with two stents sited. His regular medications were: atorvastatin 80 mg ON and aspirin 75 mg OD. The patient worked as an art teacher and lived with his wife and two teenaged children. He was an ex-smoker with a 25-pack year history and did not drink alcohol.

Examination

The patient appeared dyspnoeic but otherwise well. He was warm and well perfused. His heart rate was 180 bpm and his blood pressure was 140/90 mmHg. There was no peripheral oedema.

Results

Bloods: WCC 12.1, Hb 150, Plt 345, Na 135, K 3.7, Mg 0.78, Creat 80, CRP 23

The ECG showed a narrow complex tachycardia, consistent with a supraventricular tachycardia (this is likely to have developed secondary to dehydration).

Question

Following three vagal manoeuvres with failure to revert to sinus rhythm, the emergency department consultant advises you to prescribe and administer intravenous adenosine. Based on the above information, select the two most appropriate statements below that should be discussed with the patient prior to administering adenosine.

He should be advised that he will receive one bolus injection of adenosine	☐
He should be advised that he will probably feel better as soon as the adenosine is administered	☐
He should be advised that he will feel more unwell as soon as the adenosine is administered	☐
He should be asked to confirm that he does not have asthma	☐
He should be asked to confirm that he does not have type 2 diabetes mellitus	☐

ANSWER

He should be advised that he will receive one bolus injection of adenosine	☐
He should be advised that he will probably feel better as soon as the adenosine is administered	☐
He should be advised that he will feel more unwell as soon as the adenosine is administered	X
He should be asked to confirm that he does not have asthma	X
He should be asked to confirm that he does not have type 2 diabetes mellitus	☐

The patient should be advised that the aim of the adenosine bolus is to 'reset' the heart and that he may develop a sense of severe panic that is often described as 'impending doom'. This sensation often develops during the brief period of heart block with transient asystole prior to restoration of sinus rhythm. Tell the patient that this will last for 3–4 s and that he should breathe slowly and deeply and the sensation will soon pass. He should also be informed that up to three bolus injections of adenosine may be required to achieve chemical cardioversion.

Adenosine should be avoided in patients with asthma and those with chronic obstructive pulmonary disease with significant bronchoconstriction. This is because adenosine can induce bronchoconstriction. Asthma was previously an absolute contraindication to adenosine use; however, recent data suggests that intravenous adenosine is a less potent bronchoconstrictor than previously thought. Asthma is now considered to be a relative contraindication to intravenous adenosine use, although inhaled adenosine is still widely accepted to be absolutely contraindicated in patients with asthma.

History

A 32-year-old man is brought to the emergency department after having a 5-min tonic clonic seizure in the street. The episode was witnessed by a passing nurse who described the patient collapsing and developing jerking movements of his arms and legs. There was associated tongue biting and urinary incontinence. The patient was post-ictal on arrival and thus unable to provide any history. He had a packet of phenytoin tablets in his bag.

Examination

The patient was drowsy and disorientated but was able to obey basic commands and was moving all four limbs. Cardiovascular, respiratory and abdominal examinations were unremarkable.

Results

Bloods: WCC 10.9, Hb 152, Plt 287, Na 138, K 3.8, Creat 74, CRP <1, phenytoin level 4 (reference range 10–20 mg/L)

Question

From the options below, please select *two* appropriate management plans:

The dose of phenytoin may need to be increased	☐
The dose of phenytoin may need to be reduced	☐
The phenytoin level is uninterpretable as dosing timings are not known	☐
You should discuss adherence to phenytoin with the patient	☐
The patient should discontinue phenytoin and use an alternate agent	☐

ANSWER

The dose of phenytoin may need to be increased	X
The dose of phenytoin may need to be reduced	☐
The phenytoin level is uninterpretable as dosing timings are not known	☐
You should discuss adherence to phenytoin with the patient	X
The patient should discontinue phenytoin and use an alternate agent	☐

Phenytoin has a narrow therapeutic index and drug levels should be checked in patients who continue to experience seizures (possible underdosing) or symptoms consistent with phenytoin toxicity (overdosing). This patient has had a seizure despite apparently being on phenytoin therapy and his phenytoin level is low. Phenytoin levels are taken immediately prior to the next dose (i.e. trough concentration); therefore, this patient's phenytoin is definitely low, regardless of the timing of his last dose.

This could indicate that the dose that he is prescribed is not high enough and needs to be titrated up. Alternatively, the patient may not be adhering to the prescribed therapy by not taking his phenytoin tablets at the appropriate frequency. The patient is likely to be able to provide more information when he is fully awake post-seizure.

Question

Of these antiepileptic drugs, identify the *two* that have dosage errors:

Carbamazepine	400 mg	PO	BD	☐
Clonazepam	60 mg	PO	OD	☐
Lamotrigine	200 mg	PO	OD	☐
Levetiracetam	500 mg	PO	OD	☐
Phenytoin	2 g	PO	OD	☐
Sodium valproate	500 mg	PO	BD	☐

ANSWER

Carbamazepine	400 mg	PO	BD	☐
Clonazepam	60 mg	PO	OD	X
Lamotrigine	200 mg	PO	OD	☐
Levetiracetam	500 mg	PO	OD	☐
Phenytoin	2 g	PO	OD	X
Sodium valproate	500 mg	PO	BD	☐

Clonazepam should be prescribed at a dose of 4–8 mg ON. Prescribers frequently confuse clonazepam with clobazam, which is dosed at 20–30 mg OD, up to a maximum of 60 mg OD.

Phenytoin is dosed at 200–500 mg daily orally. The intravenous loading dose of phenytoin (as used in status epilepticus) is 20 mg/kg (maximum dose 2 g).

History

A 45-year-old woman was admitted to hospital (day 0) with a 5-day history of worsening right iliac fossa pain. She was diagnosed with a ruptured appendix and underwent an appendicectomy. The following day (day 1), she developed shortness of breath and left-sided chest pain on deep inspiration. A CT pulmonary angiogram showed a left-sided subsegmental pulmonary embolus. The patient was prescribed an unfractionated heparin infusion due to her significant bleeding risk and potential need for further abdominal surgery.

Examination

The patient appears comfortable at rest and is awake and alert. Her abdomen is soft with right iliac fossa tenderness. Her wound appears clean and dry. Her heart sounds are normal with no murmurs. Her heart rate is 100 bpm and her blood pressure is 98/50 mmHg.

Results

Day 0 – platelet count 350×10^9
Day 2 – platelet count 362×10^9
Day 3 – platelet count 348×10^9
Day 4 – platelet count 301×10^9
Day 5 – platelet count 270×10^9
Day 6 – platelet count 150×10^9
Day 7 – platelet count 90×10^9

Question

Based on the above results, which *one* of the management options below would be most appropriate?

Continue heparin infusion and monitor for signs of bleeding	☐
Increase the rate of the heparin infusion	☐
Stop heparin infusion and give no further anti-coagulant therapy at present	☐
Stop heparin infusion and commence enoxaparin 1.5 mg/kg SC	☐
Stop heparin infusion and commence fondaparinux 7.5 mg SC	☐

ANSWER

Continue heparin infusion and monitor for signs of bleeding	☐
Increase the rate of the heparin infusion	☐
Stop heparin infusion and give no further anti-coagulant therapy at present	☐
Stop heparin infusion and commence enoxaparin 1.5 mg/kg SC	☐
Stop heparin infusion and commence fondaparinux 7.5 mg SC	X

The patient is likely to have developed heparin-induced thrombocytopaenia (HIT). This typically develops 4–5 days after commencing heparin treatment. HIT typically develops after exposure to unfractionated heparin and is far less common in patients receiving low molecular weight heparins.

The patient has a pulmonary embolism and needs to continue on an anticoagulant therapy. Additionally, HIT is a pro-coagulant state despite the low platelet count. She should be treated with fondaparinux now – this is a low molecular weight heparin that is often used to anticoagulate patients who have developed HIT as it has a comparatively low affinity for platelet factor 4 and is less likely to induce HIT compared with other heparins.

History

A 65-year-old man presented to his general practitioner for a routine review. He had been feeling well over recent weeks. His past medical history included hypertension and hypercholesterolaemia. His regular medications were amlodipine 10 mg OD and atorvastatin 20 mg ON. He had no known drug allergies or intolerances. He was a retired shopkeeper and lived with his partner. He was an ex-smoker with a 20-pack year history and he drank approximately 10 units of alcohol per week.

Examination

The patient appeared generally well. His heart rate was 70 bpm and his blood pressure was 160/88 mmHg. His heart sounds were dual with no murmurs. There was no peripheral oedema. Systems examination was otherwise unremarkable.

Results

Bloods: WCC 8.8, Hb 149, Plt 320, Na 140, K 4.0, Creat 67

Question

Which *one* of the options below would be the most appropriate management plan for this patient?

Add in doxazosin 4 mg OD	☐
Add in indapamide (modified release) 1.5 mg PO OD	☐
Add in ramipril 2.5 mg PO OD	☐
Continue on his current medications	☐

ANSWER

Add in doxazosin 4 mg OD	☐
Add in indapamide (modified release) 1.5 mg PO OD	☐
Add in ramipril 2.5 mg PO OD	X
Continue on his current medications	☐

In patients with essential hypertension, the National Institute for Health and Care Excellence (NICE) recommend that adults over the age of 55 years should commence a calcium channel blocker as the first-line antihypertensive. The next agent to be added in is either an angiotensin converting enzyme (ACE) inhibitor or an angiotensin II type 1 receptor blocker (ARB). Ramipril is, therefore, the correct agent in this scenario. The third-line drug to be added in is typically a thiazide-like diuretic, such as indapamide (Figure 99.1).

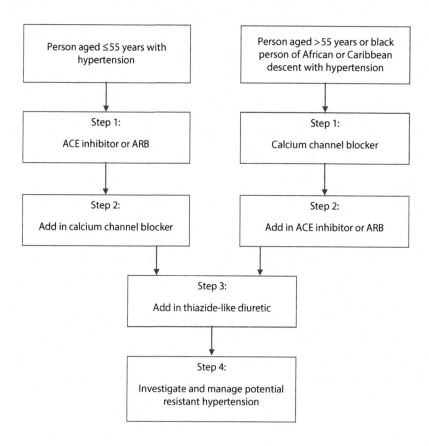

Figure 99.1 Management steps for essential hypertension.

Question

Of the drugs given below, identify the *two* that have dosage errors:

Atorvastatin	40 mg	PO	ON	☐
Chlorphenamine	40 mg	PO	OD	☐
Clonidine	50 mg	PO	TDS	☐
Cyclizine	50 mg	PO	TDS	☐
Metoclopramide	10 mg	PO	TDS	☐
Omeprazole	20 mg	PO	OD	☐
Promethazine	20 mg	PO	OD	☐

ANSWER

Atorvastatin	40 mg	PO	ON	☐
Chlorphenamine	40 mg	PO	OD	X
Clonidine	50 mg	PO	TDS	X
Cyclizine	50 mg	PO	TDS	☐
Metoclopramide	10 mg	PO	TDS	☐
Omeprazole	20 mg	PO	OD	☐
Promethazine	20 mg	PO	OD	☐

Chlorphenamine is an antihistamine that is typically prescribed at doses of 4 mg every 4–6 h up to a maximum 24 mg per day.

Clonidine is an α-adrenergic agent that is prescribed in the treatment of hypertension. Clonidine is prescribed at a dose of 50–100 µg (not milligrams) three times a day, titrating up to a maximum dose 1.2 mg daily.

INDEX

Note: Page numbers in italic and bold refer to figures and tables, respectively.